THE INFLAMMATORY DIET GUIDE

Complete Beginner's Guide To Fight Inflammation, Heal The Immune System And Live A Healthier Life

ELIZABETH WELLS

Copyright © 2018 Elizabeth Wells

All rights reserved.

In no way is it legal to reproduce, duplicate, or transmit any part of this document in either electronic means or in printed format. recording of this publication is strictly prohibited and any storage of this document is not allowed unless with written permission from the publisher. all rights reserved. The information provided herein is stated to be truthful and consistent, in that any liability, in terms of inattention or otherwise, by any usage or abuse of any policies, processes, or directions contained within is the solitary and utter responsibility of the recipient reader. under no circumstances will any legal responsibility or blame be held against the publisher for any reparation, damages, or monetary loss due to the information herein, either directly or indirectly. Respective authors own all copyrights not held by the publisher. The information herein is offered for informational purposes solely, and is universal as so. the presentation of the information is without contract or any type of guarantee assurance. The trademarks that are used are without any consent, and the publication of the trademark is without permission or backing by the trademark owner. all trademarks and brands within this book are for clarifying purposes only and are the owned by the owners themselves, not affiliated with this document. The author wishes to thank rez_art / 123RF for the image on the cover.

TABLE OF CONTENTS

Free Bonus: The Best Foods To Eat On A Ketogenic Diet..........................7

Introduction..9

Chapter 1: Inflammation..12

Chapter 2: Anti-Inflammatory Diet - Path to Good Health.....................17

Chapter 3: Are You Suffering From Any Of These?................................24

Chapter 4: Common Myths About Anti-Inflammatory Diet....................35

Chapter 5: The Ways to Make Your Anti-Inflammatory Diet Awesome..40

Chapter 6: Food Items to Include In Your Anti-Inflammatory Diet..........43

Chapter 7: The Plan to Get the Best from Your Anti-Inflammatory Diet.76

Chapter 8: Foods to Avoid For a Healthy Body..81

Conclusion..86

Other Books By Elizabeth Wells..89

Free Bonus

The Best Foods To Eat On A Ketogenic Diet

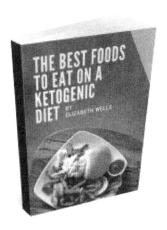

Discover the best foods to eat on a ketogenic diet. You'll learn the different food groups that you should eat to follow the keto diet correctly and start improving your health right now.

Go to **www.eepurl.com/cUqOlH** to download the guide for free.

Introduction

Congratulations on purchasing this book and thank you for doing so.

Excess of anything is bad, and inflammation is a classic example of this. It demonstrates how a good thing can start working against you if it doesn't remain in check. Inflammation in concept is your body's defense mechanism to prevent damage. It is the repair mechanism. But, when the damage is persistent, this mechanism goes into overdrive. It starts causing more harm to you than good, and we call it chronic inflammation. If you develop chronic inflammation, then it can cause a score of dangerous things ranging from obesity and heart diseases to even cancer.

This book will educate you about the need to have an anti-inflammatory diet. It will throw light on the problems chronic inflammation can cause and the role a bad diet plays in it. It will discuss in detail the food items you must include in your diet to avoid chronic inflammation.

Chapter 1 will explain the concept of inflammation to you. It will tell you how chronic inflammation can lead to various diseases. It will also discuss the common symptoms and main reasons for chronic inflammation.

In chapter 2 you will get to know the importance of an anti-inflammatory diet. It will discuss in detail the positive impact a good diet can have on your overall health.

Chapter 3 will tell you the main diseases that are caused by chronic inflammation. It will try to explain in detail the impact of inflammation on these illnesses. This chapter will open your eyes about the misconceptions we have been having about some illnesses and their causes.

The 4th Chapter will bust some of the common myths about an anti-inflammatory diet. Ignorance is among the greatest evils as it makes you trust even baseless facts. This chapter clears the misconception about anti-inflammatory diet so that you can accept it with an open heart. People usually put stickers tasteless or bland to any good diet. This chapter clears the air about it.

Chapter 5 will tell you some ways in which you can spice up your anti-inflammatory diet and make it savory and soulful. It tells you the healthy ways to get a taste.

Chapter 6 will explain in detail the food items you must include in your anti-inflammatory diet. It is a comprehensive chapter will a wide list of food items that you can include. You will not feel short of good things to eat.

Chapter 7 will tell you the diet plan you must have and the things you must consume on a regular basis.

The chapter 8 will discuss the food items you must

avoid to remain healthy. It will also explain the problems they cause so that you always remain informed.

This book is a descriptive guide to good health. It will open your mind about the advantages of having a good diet and the positive impact it can have on your life. Food is a very important part of our lives. We cannot ignore it. We all want to have a good diet but most never follow it due to lack of information. This book clears the air and makes your choice of good health easy for you.

You will have plenty of food items to choose from so that you can remain healthy. Chronic inflammation can have serious repercussions, and this book will explain in detail how it affects your health. It will also tell you how you can avoid chronic inflammation and reduce the risk of diseases caused by chronic inflammation.

There are plenty of books on this subject on the market, thanks again for choosing this one! Every effort was made to ensure it is full of as much useful information as possible, please enjoy!

Chapter 1
Inflammation

What is Inflammation?

Inflammation is a normal occurrence. You bang your knee somewhere, it swells and become red in that area. You eat something very hot and spicy and upset your stomach. You sleep in a wrong posture and wake up with stiffness in limbs. These are all responses from your body. The body is trying to repair itself to get things back to normal. These reactions are Inflammation.

In simple terms, inflammation is not a disease. It is our body's response mechanism to outside invasion of germs and infections.

Your body is a fort, and it is in hot pursuit. Germs and infections are trying to capture this fort. Your body's defense mechanism fights well. It protects you from regular infections. Inflammation is a signal that damage control is going on in specific parts. It uses a lot of energy. You may start feeling weak and tired during inflammation. This is normal. There isn't much to worry about in normal circumstances. A fever is an inflammation to fight the invasion of germs. Tenderness and swelling in wounds help in repairing skin and tissue damage. Upset bowel movement or acid refluxes may be an indicator that some germs have attacked your gut. Your body can counter most of these issues without much external help.

Take Note of Regular Inflammations

If these issues arise once in a while and go away in a short span, then your immune system is working great. However, if you are experiencing these issues very often and they are taking a toll on your health, then you must get alert. Your immune system may be caving in, and it might be asking for help. A healthy lifestyle and a well-balanced anti-inflammatory diet can do the trick for you. Your immune system will get the required help.

Inflammation is a sign that the body is facing an attack of infections. It is a plea for reinforcement and help. Our immune system can fight infections, but it will not win without help. No one can fight without aid forever.

Chronic Inflammation is Bad

Inflammation raises many red flags. It is important that you take note of them and start taking corrective steps while still there is time to do so. Delay can cause chronic infections and serious diseases.

To bring things into perspective consider these important facts:

1. Unattended inflammation in the joints can lead to Rheumatoid arthritis and Psoriatic arthritis.

2. Inflammation of kidneys may lead to high blood pressure and even kidney failure.

3. Inflammation of heart can cause shortness of breath and may also lead to fluid retention.

4. Early signs of aging and wrinkles are also a result of recurring inflammations.

The list of such problems is endless. Long-term inflammations may also lead to asthma, peptic ulcer, tuberculosis, and even some types of cancers. It is important to manage inflammations well. Unattended inflammation can do more harm than good. It is your body's call for help. You need to understand the distress call and pay heed to it.

What Causes Inflammation?

Germs like bacteria, virus, and fungi are the most common cause of Inflammation. However, inflammation can also occur due to injuries like scrapes and wounds. Chemical and radiation effects can also lead to inflammation.

Common Symptoms

The common symptoms of acute inflammation are redness, heat, swelling, pain, loss of sensation in specific areas. At times, there may not be any symptom of inflammation. Your body may curb the infections on its own. It is very important to note that inflammation is a response to infections. The immune system works very hard. But, it needs to be supplemented. If it keeps facing such attacks but doesn't get any outside help, then the infections will win, and you may fall sick.

3 Main Reasons for Recurring Inflammations

Environmental Factors

In the current environmental scenario, the air we breathe in is highly polluted. The food we eat is contaminated with pesticides, herbicides, and metals. The water available at most places is also adulterated. The immune system is not getting any outside help. In fact, these things are weakening it to a great extent.

Stressful Life

To add salt to the injury, the increasing stress in life further aggravates the problems. Higher stress creates an imbalance in our pH levels. This prepares a favorable ground for bad bacteria to flourish and may lead to recurring inflammation and diseases.

Unhealthy Food and Lifestyle Choices

Apart from all this, the final blow comes from the diet and lifestyle we adopt. Too much fast food is a big problem. It is laden with a lot of sugar and unsaturated fats. They are a big problem. Too much of caffeine and carbonated drinks also weaken our system. If you have a sedentary lifestyle, then you will be prone to inflammation. Erratic sleep cycles may also cause problems. These are some of the things that aid and abet inflammation.

You Must Never Ignore Inflammation

Inflammation may not seem to be a big problem to you, but it is definitely not a problem that can be ignored. It is a sign that your body is fighting a losing battle. If you do not act fast, then it will surrender. The result would not only come in the form of diseases and infections, but you can also see visible signs of aging and wrinkles as a result of inflammation.

Recurring Inflammation can be Dangerous

If you contract bacterial, viral and fungal infections

regularly, then it may be a result of inflammation. It can also lead to acid refluxes and stomach related problems. Negligence of chronic inflammation may lead to the development of serious health issues too. Lifestyle diseases like diabetes, blood pressure, and heart diseases are common.

You cannot take inflammation lightly. Adopting preventive measures is the best option. The best thing is that it isn't very difficult. Adoption of an anti-inflammatory diet and a healthy lifestyle can help you in strengthening your immune system. It will help you in preventing inflammations from getting chronic.

Chapter 2
Anti-Inflammatory Diet - Path to Good Health

We understand that normal inflammation is not a scary scenario. But, this doesn't mean that it isn't taxing for your immune system. Your immune system has to work overtime. You can do a big favor to your immune system by adopting a diet that provides some help. Before we proceed any further on this topic, it is important to understand how this can help anyway.

Gut Health is Very Important

Gut health is of great importance for your immune system. More than 80 percent of your immune system is in your gut. If you keep on eating inflammatory food, then the immune system takes a severe hit. You can get prone to inflammations.

Help Your Immune System through Diet

Besides this, to fight regular infections your immune system needs regular assistance. This can come in a form of vitamin and minerals from your anti-inflammatory diet. The correct diet plays a very important role in your health. If you consume inflammatory foods, your body would need to overwork. It will face a shortage of adequate supplies. Irritable bowel symptoms, achy joints, bloating, various allergies, puffiness are very common issues. We face them in our day-to-day lives but never pay attention to the cause. In most of the cases, intake of inflammatory foods is the root cause of these problems. Inflammatory food can not only cause health issues but may also lead to mental exhaustion and anxiety. Unhealthy gut function and depression have a direct connection.

Open the Doors to a Healthy Life

An Anti-Inflammatory Diet has several advantages. It will help you in leading a healthy and happy life. It uplifts your physical, mental and emotional well-being. There is an old saying 'we become what we eat.' It holds true in every respect. The food we eat has a great impact on us. If we adopt dietary habits that are calming and do not irritate our immune system, then we will be able to lead a healthier and happier life.

8 Remarkable Benefits of Adopting an Anti-Inflammatory Diet:

1. Get Your Glow Back

Regular inflammations have a direct impact on the health of the skin. After all, skin is the largest organ in your body. If you are prone to inflammation or have any chronic inflammation, then it will show up on your skin. Dullness, acne, blemishes, itchiness, and rashes are some of the common effects. Recurring inflammation can have a deep impact on the glow of your skin. It can make your skin dull and lackluster.

You must avoid inflammatory foods like sugar, yeast,

gluten, soy and dairy products.

Anti-inflammatory food rich in vitamins, minerals, and antioxidants can revitalize your skin. It will help your immune system in fighting infections and also help your skin regain the lost glow from within.

2. Make Weight Loss a Reality

It is a no-brainer that some foods lead to excess gain weight and make shedding the extra pounds very difficult. The problem doesn't stop only at gaining some extra pounds. Inflammation of fat cells can wreak havoc on its victims. It may lead to insulin resistance in future, making weight loss very tough. The inflammation of cells in other organs like the brain can lead to metabolic disorders.

Obesity and diabetes have a close relationship. One generally leads to the other. Systematic inflammation is a scary scenario, and you must try to avoid it. Exclusion of food products containing corn, gluten, soy, yeast, and dairy items will help in decreasing the chances of allergies and inflammation.

You can easily lose weight by adopting a planned anti-inflammatory diet and following an active lifestyle. It doesn't need to remain a distant dream anymore.

3. Boost Your Brain Power

Mental well-being has a direct relation to physical well-being. To have a peaceful mind, you need to have a stable constitution. Chronic inflammation can prove to be a great impediment to this. It can push you towards depression, anxiety, mental exhaustion, and indecisiveness. If you have been experiencing the foggy start of the day with blurred thoughts or mood swings, then you immediately need attention. Frequent zoning out, mental fatigue and regular loss of focus can be a result of chronic inflammation. Poor diet has a direct connection with this condition.

Our brain is the most vital organ in our body, and its integrity is very important. Several studies have proved that poor gut function, chronic inflammation, and depression have a direct link. An anti-inflammatory diet rich in phytonutrients and antioxidants can give your brain the much-needed help.

4. Give Your Gut the Needed Respite

The busy lifestyle of this fast-paced world has tailored us to treat our gut as a dustbin. We throw whatever we manage to get to fill it up. Seldom do we care about the quality of the food we pull up. It is not due to the scarcity of time or money but the sheer carelessness. The result we face is in the form of bloating, constipation, diarrhea, and acidity. The main cause of these problems is the microbial imbalance in the gut known as Gut Dysbiosis.

Our gut has hundreds of species of good and bad bacteria that help in the digestion of food. The balance helps in fighting several infections too. But, inconsiderate intake of food items can toss it for a spin. This may lead to serious consequences. Damage to the gut lining, irritable bowel disease, and leaky gut are some of the diseases that can occur.

Apart from these long-term impacts, you can feel constant discomfort, puffy stomach, loss of appetite and other similar issues.

Intake of anti-inflammatory diet along with probiotics is the easiest way to resolve these issues.

A good diet takes less effort and money. It only needs the desire to do the right things correctly.

5. Get Over Joint Pain

Joint pain is simply debilitating. It literally brings you to your knees. Every step in life becomes excruciatingly painful, and there is no going back. Surgery may give you momentary relief, but you know that nothing feels as good as the original. Chronic inflammation of joints can lead to such condition. People suffering from such condition need to take tons of medication, and yet the relief is just a consolation. Cutting down on sugar and gluten along with anti-inflammatory diet can prove to be a miracle for such people.

A change in diet can bring a revolutionary change in the life of people suffering from joint pain and related issues like arthritis.

6. Get Control Over Cravings

We all are puppets of desire. Yet, not being able to control some cravings can spell a lot of trouble. Excess intake of artificial sweeteners and refined sugar can start a vicious cycle of craving and inflammation. It will not only lead to piling up of excess weight, but you will also get chronic inflammation.

Once this cycle starts, things start spiraling out of your control. The urge to eat more sweets takes precedence over your rational thinking. The right way to break it is to adopt a planned anti-inflammatory diet. Intake of the correct ingredients at regular intervals will not only curb your urge to eat more, but it will also add healthy nutrients to your body.

7. Burn Excess Fat

Everyone dreams of having an admirable physique and bulging tires of fat do not fit that description. Excess fat is not only a cosmetic problem, but it also creates a very unhealthy situation. Excess accumulation of fat has a direct link with inflammation. In case of chronic inflammation, the fat cells get infected. The body sends a hormone by the name Leptin to the brain to indicate fullness, and you lose your appetite. In case of inflammation, the message never gets conveyed and your craving to eat more persists.

This leads to intake of more fat than you can consume and hence the accumulation takes place.

This Leptin resistance is one of the biggest factors responsible for the problem. Intake of trans fat, polyunsaturated fats, vegetable oils and partially hydrogenated oils lead to the problem.

Anti-inflammatory diet not only eliminates these oils from your food but it also cuts down sugar and other harmful ingredients. Introduction of helpful fats along with the ingredients that positive nutrients will help in controlling your craving for food. You will not only burn fat faster but will also be able to control your blood sugar levels.

8. Much Needed Relief from Allergies

Allergies are a big nuisance. They lead us to days of isolation. Incessant sneezing, runny nose, itchy eyes, and headaches are some of the problems caused by allergies. Allergies are no fun to anyone, and they are unbearable for most. However, seasonal allergies can be avoided to a great extent by making the right changes in the diet. You need to remove the items that irritate your gut. Bananas, yeast, wines, pickles, fish, food additives, artificial sweeteners are some of the items that aggravate allergies. You will need to remove these items from your diet to get relief. The focus must be towards decreasing the inflammation of the gut. It is the area where most of the problems originate.

An anti-inflammatory diet can put you on the path to good health. It will make you energetic and lively. It only needs your intent and determination.

Chapter 3
Are You Suffering From Any Of These?

In this chapter, we will discuss some diseases which can make lives of the sufferers a living hell. We will also discuss how adopting an inflammatory diet can help with those problems. This chapter will try to open you up towards the miraculous impact of anti-inflammatory diet in real life.

Diabetes

Diabetes is a defeating disease. It can pull down even the most towering individuals. Although it is mostly believed to be a genetic disorder, the fact that it is also a lifestyle disorder. Obesity and inactivity are the main culprits that can lead to diabetes. Apart from these, the other most common reason for diabetes is chronic inflammation.

It is now an established fact that long-term inflammation in fat cells can lead to insulin resistance. Acute inflammations are easily detected and treated. But, low-grade inflammation goes undetected and keeps working behind the scene. It can build up over a period of time and can cause long-term problems like diabetes, obesity, and heart diseases.

Various studies have demonstrated that anti-inflammatory diet can help you stay safe. The toughest part in stopping this kind of diabetes is that you don't even know about it till it has arrived. By that time, it gets very late. An anti-inflammatory diet can help in keeping low-grade chronic infections at bay. It will also help you in keeping the obesity in check.

Anti-inflammatory foods containing omega-3 fatty acids like the flaxseed oil, olive oil, canola oil, avocados, walnuts, fruits, and vegetable are very helpful. Glucose in fruits isn't harmful and helps in regulating blood glucose. It also helps in stopping inflammation. Antioxidants, omega-3, and fiber-rich diet can be your answer to the low-grade chronic inflammation that silently keeps on building up.

Obesity

Some studies prove that some obesity-inducing genetic factors get activated by inflammatory diet. The diet-induced low-level chronic inflammation helps in the accumulation of excess weight. It can have serious metabolic consequences. Unfortunately, we have increased the consumption of refined carbohydrates, vegetable oils, and omega-6 fatty acids. Our intake of omega-3 fatty acids, which is the most beneficial nutrient for us, has decreased. This has created a great imbalance, and the obesity-inducing genes have got a free ride.

Inflammatory foods are harmful in many ways. They not only lead to accumulation of excess weight but also agitate our immune system. Prolonged inflammation in the fat cells creates further complications. The production of appetite-regulating hormones gets affected, and the body loses control of food regulation. You start eating as much as you want. This all eventually leads to excess weight gain. You gain weight because you are eating more, and you keep on eating more. This is a vicious cycle.

Anti-inflammatory food helps you in breaking this vicious cycle. It suppresses your urge to eat more while fulfilling your energy needs. It provides relief from the inflammation and heals you from inside. Low-level chronic inflammation is very difficult to diagnose and treat. By the time you get to know about it, the critical time has already passed. The correct diet helps you in checking it.

An anti-inflammatory diet for obesity should be full of whole nutrient dense foods that contain antioxidants. You must avoid processed products as a rule. Your every meal should have a good balance of protein, carbs, and fat. You must get the required minerals, vitamins, fiber and water. An anti-inflammatory diet is not about starving yourself, but it is about fulfilling your energy needs in a stable and sensible way.

Fresh green leafy vegetables, berries, high-fat fruits, healthy fats, fatty fish, nuts, peppers, and spices are some of the ingredients of an anti-inflammatory diet.

Heart Diseases

Cholesterol, publicly defamed as the villain of most of the heart diseases doesn't lead to heart diseases by itself. The actual culprit is the inflammation that leads to oxidation of cholesterol particles. An anti-inflammatory diet rich in antioxidants can help you in slowing or curbing this process. It is important to note that oxidative stress plays a key role in heart diseases. Omega-3 fatty acids have anti-inflammatory properties that slow down this process. Foods rich in antioxidants, polyunsaturated fatty acids and vitamins C and E can also be very helpful.

Studies have proven that carotenoids and vitamin C and E lower the risk of heart diseases. Consumption of fish rich in polyunsaturated fatty acids also lowers the risk of heart diseases and strokes. Natural products like fruits and vegetables have a very beneficial impact on the functioning of the heart.

A diet rich in high-quality fresh fruits and vegetables, unrefined cereals, olive oil, nuts, legumes, yogurt, and fish can work wonders for the heart. Intake of meat, eggs, sweets, and alcohol must be cut down. The stress should be on eating fresh fruits and vegetables. Processed foods spell great danger for your heart, and they must be avoided as much as possible.

Your heart works very hard. You can stress it more by consuming inflammatory food items. It would still work for some time but wouldn't last for more. Do not overburden an already hardworking organ. Help it by eating food rich in antioxidants, omega-3 fatty acids, polyunsaturated fat, and fiber.

Heart diseases have become a major reason for deaths in the US. As per the recent statistics, one out of four deaths took place due to heart diseases. The risk is big, and the solution is in front of you. You can either choose to face the problem with a solution or just duck away and keep feigning as if the problem never existed in the first place. The former will take you towards a healthy and fulfilling life, and the latter wouldn't take you anywhere at all. The road ahead is short and painful.

Choosing a healthy anti-inflammatory diet is easy and beneficial. You only need to see the long-term benefits and work towards adopting it.

Cancer

Cancer has a deadly and frightening tone to it. Only its mention can send a chill down the spine of people. It is scary not only to those people who faced cancer or have had cancer victims in their circle but also to those people who have just heard of it. Yet, the presence and imminent danger of cancer is a harsh reality.

Chronic inflammation has a direct link with many types of cancers. Inflammatory response stimulates our immune system to start acting on specific parts of our body. Chronic inflammation can confuse the sensors that stop this process. It can lead to overproduction or unregulated production of cells. The problem is that such chronic inflammations do not show any visible signs. They keep agitating the system stealthily sending the immune system into overdrive. Several diseases like Crohn's disease, Inflammatory Bowel Syndrome, esophagitis, hepatitis, etc., can turn into various types of cancers. The longer it takes to control the inflammation, the higher are the chances of developing cancer.

Inflammatory foods can have a deep impact on this. Such foods provide triggers to inflammation and keep flaring it up. To reduce the risk, it is important that you put a stop on this or at least reduce it to safer levels.

Anti-inflammatory foods have a very important role to play here. Systematic identification of the inflammation-triggering foods and their elimination from your diet can be of great help. Intake of food products that are soothing and provide the healing elements can even help in faster recovery. Chronic inflammations are hard to cure through medication as they lie low. But, intake of anti-inflammatory food can have a great impact on them.

It can cure your inflammation fast and stop it from developing into cancer. Once any cancer has developed, such a diet can help you in recovering fast and leading a healthy life.

Anti-inflammatory diet would be based on the kind of problem you are facing and the inflammatory triggers you have. Careful planning and elimination of the agitating elements will play a very important role in the diet.

Rheumatoid Arthritis (RA)

Rheumatoid Arthritis is a perfect example of our own immune system going into overdrive. It is a very painful condition where the joints hurt badly. The lining of the joints get affected, and this causes immense pain during the movement of the limbs. The inflammation of joints can also lead to bone erosion and joint deformity.

This is a chronic illness and lasts for the lifetime. Once in its grip, the patient has no avenue for escape. Anti-inflammatory diet has shown a ray of hope to the people suffering from Rheumatoid Arthritis. This diet can ease up the inflammation and provide great relief.

Some foods items like gluten, corn, dairy products, processed sugar, soy, and alcohol can trigger inflammation. Consuming them can make your life really difficult. You will have to avoid them at all costs or else even the medications wouldn't have that great effect.

On the other hand, several food items can really ease your pain. Food items that are rich in Omega-3 fatty acids and Vitamin D are really helpful. You can get plenty of them from fatty fish varieties like Salmon and trout.

Ginger and garlic are two items that work wonders in relieving pain in RA. They contain anti-inflammatory properties and decrease the levels of inflammatory markers in the body. Broccoli, walnuts, berries, spinach, grapes, and olive oil are some other items that are rich in Omega-3 fatty acids, antioxidants, vitamin D, monosaturated fats, protein, and fiber.

A balanced diet comprising these food items can help you in relieving the symptoms of RA and to enjoy your life.

Psoriasis

Most people do not consider dandruff or discolored skin to be a serious problem. Some can even take sensitive, itchy and painful lesions as a non-threatening issue. However, for the victims of Psoriasis, these symptoms are a big problem. Psoriasis is just not a cosmetic problem. It is painful and has high susceptibility to turn into psoriatic arthritis.

Some of the main reasons for psoriasis are an overactive immune system, poor diet, a leaky gut and difficulty in digesting protein.

Probiotic foods like kefir, yogurt, and apple cider vinegar can help in reducing inflammation and increasing immunity. High-fiber food is also great for such a condition. Antioxidant-rich foods like fruits, vegetables, herbs, beans, and nuts also provide great relief. The people suffering from such a condition should also increase the intake of foods rich in zinc and vitamin A.

Psoriasis is an autoimmune disorder, and hence the medication can only have a limited impact. The best way to get relief is to adopt an anti-inflammatory diet, exercise and drink plenty of water.

Some foods such as fatty red meats can really cause great trouble for the patients. These contain very high levels of cholesterol and saturated fats and hence give rise to blood sugar. Choosing leaner proteins is the best choice. Processed foods and refined sugar should also be avoided.

Food sources rich in protein and low in saturated fats are especially good. Coldwater fish like mackerel, salmon, herring and lake trout are really good for this. They are also a rich source of Omega-3 fatty acids. Flax seeds, olive oils, pumpkin seeds, and walnuts are also great for such condition. Colorful fresh fruits and vegetables are also very helpful.

Asthma

Asthma can be life-threatening. Even when it doesn't keep the patients tied to the line. The restrictions are immense, and there is always a fear. The worst part is that it is a chronic disease. There is no proper cure for asthma, and the patients have to bear with it. Taking precautions, avoiding unnecessary health risks and a balanced anti-inflammatory diet is important.

The occurrence of asthma has risen considerably in the past few decades, and researchers believe that poor food habits are responsible for it to a great extent. Lower intake of fresh fruits and vegetable and a greater shift towards processed foods may have led to it. Several studies have concluded that intake of food items rich in vitamin C & E, beta-carotene, and flavonoids lower the risks of contracting asthma. Magnesium, selenium and omega-3 fatty acids play an important role in relieving its symptoms. Taking an antioxidant-rich diet is the key here. This will prevent cell damage, and the patients will feel better.

Trans fats and omega-6 fatty acids must be avoided at all costs. They can spell trouble by worsening the condition and may also lead to other health conditions such as heart diseases. Asthma patients should also avoid high-calorie diets as they may lead to excess weight gain. Allergic food items must always be kept away.

Fighting asthma can be tiresome. It is a condition that keeps you on your toes at all times. The best way to deal with it is to have a healthy lifestyle. Incorporate a healthy diet to stay safe and keep a distance from allergic things.

Esophagitis

Esophagitis is an inflammation-driven problem. Its common symptoms include abdominal pain, difficulty in swallowing, heartburn, and mouth sores. If not treated properly and in a timely manner, it can cause serious damage to the esophagus, the food pipe.

As discussed earlier, the main cause of esophagitis is inflammation. Avoiding allergic foods and things which could lead to inflammatory response is the most helpful. GERD or acid reflux in simple terms is the most common cause of esophagitis. If you can control gut inflammation, then its occurrence can be minimized. Allergic items can flare up inflammation in the esophagus, and hence they must be avoided. If you are allergic to certain food products, then you should eliminate them from your diet.

The people suffering from this problem can have a very hard time while eating. A cough, nausea, vomiting, and difficulty in swallowing solid foods is a common complaint.

Food that is low in fat and high in protein is very helpful. Spicy, fatty and acidic food must be avoided. The focus must be towards eating things that do not cause acidity or allergy. Eating small meals and eating at small intervals is also a good way to avoid acidity that can aggravate the problem.

Alcohol, caffeine and carbonated beverages must be eliminated from the diet. Easy to digest fruits like banana, peeled apples, pears are a good choice. Fruits and vegetables that are rich in vitamins, minerals, and fiber must be included in the diet plan. The main focus should be on reducing the inflammation.

Crohn's Disease

Inflammation of the lining of your digestive tract can give birth to Crohn's disease. It is a painful and debilitating condition. It can make the life of its victims really difficult, thus reducing the quality of life. The digestive tract gets infected, and the patient may experience abdominal pain, severe diarrhea, weight loss, fatigue, and malnutrition. In some cases, this disease can become life-threatening too. In this disease, often the small intestine gets infected, and this leads to compromised absorption of nutrients. So, apart from the pain and discomfort, malnutrition also becomes a big problem. Some foods can specifically trigger the symptoms and cause problems.

An anti-inflammatory diet has a very positive impact on the patients. Change in diet and lifestyle can give great relief and the victims suffering from Crohn's disease will be able to enjoy life in a better way.

One of the main problems with diets plans for Crohn's disease is that they need to be prepared as per the needs of the individual. Some foods might trigger inflammation in your intestines while they may work for others. So each food item needs to be tested one by one. Low residue diets work well for most of the people as they help in limiting the bowel movement. Liquid diets work wonders for some people suffering from Crohn's disease. The main idea must always be to take up a diet plan that reduces inflammation in the intestines. It must also provide a high dosage of nutrients as malnutrition always remains a big problem.

Salmons, eggs, almond milk, vegetable soups, avocados, orange sweet potatoes, and yogurt are good. These foods provide the required nutrients without taxing the system.

Chapter 4
Common Myths About Anti-Inflammatory Diet

Myths are part and parcel of our lives. As soon as something picks up a pace, people start making assumptions and deductions based on their knowledge, which, for the most part of it is insufficient. The same has happened with the anti-inflammatory diet. People simply take it for granted that a dish that is to be healthy will be tasteless. It must be very costly and may require lots of your time. Your whole life will revolve around it, and you'd have nothing better to do than that. These are reasonable deductions yet, they're nowhere even close to being the truth.

Apart from the health angle, we generally weigh food on three main parameters, namely, taste, price and preparation time. In this chapter, we will discuss these factors and understand where the anti-inflammatory food stands on these scales.

A Word to the Wise

Before we proceed further, we have to classify the users into 2 groups. One, those are currently suffering from health issues related to inflammation. Two, who aren't suffering from such issues but want to adopt a healthy diet for a safe future. The former group may feel awkward in the beginning. It is normal as their transition has to be fast. It is propelled by need. They may take some time to adjust to this diet and habit.

The latter group will have a very easy time. The first reason is that they are opting this for a healthy life. They already know that health needs some sacrifices. Second, they will have the liberty to take their own time, and there is no strict curfew on cheat streaks. However, once they get accustomed to this diet, they wouldn't want to. Nothing is lacking in this diet.

An anti-inflammatory diet can be equally tasty, interesting, quick and full of variety. There is no reason for it to be boring or bland. The purpose of this diet is not to make your life difficult but to make it easy.

Some of the common MYTHS about anti-inflammatory diet are:

It will have NO taste

Nothing can be farther from the truth. Shifting to an anti-inflammatory diet is a big shift, but it doesn't need to be a painful one. You can eat most of the ingredients. Only processed sugar and saturated and trans fats are to be avoided. This doesn't take away the taste of the ingredients. You can add sweetness to the food through natural sweeteners like honey, rice malt syrups, and fruit juices. You can use healthy oils like olive oil.

The purpose of the diet is to provide you the required nutrients without causing inflammation. As long as the products are not causing inflammation or stimulating something nasty, you are free to eat them.

There are numerous recipes to make your anti-inflammatory diet lip-smackingly tasty. As a bonus, you wouldn't have those guilt trips of consuming harmful food that may hurt you later. The deal is sweeter than you have guessed.

It will cost TOO much

It will not cost more than the cost of the treatment if you are facing inflammation regularly. However, there is some truth in the fact that anti-inflammatory diet may cost you more than the processed food you eat. This being a part truth, which is a more dangerous thing. It is somewhat natural for the cost of anti-inflammatory diet to be a bit high when you are buying fresh, natural products. They will cost you more than they would have cost the companies which buy them for bulk processing. But, they are not going to cost you exorbitantly more. The difference in the pricing is mild. Community Supported Agriculture and several other models give you access to fresh fruits, vegetable and meat at a reasonable price. There is a vast difference in the taste of a fresh product and a processed one. You can actually feel the difference in the nutrition offered.

You must consider the fact that an inflammatory diet is dragging you towards health issues. In the end, you will have to spend on medications too. Even if we leave aside the dangers of chronic inflammation, the costs of treatment will be high.

Preparing such food will COST time

This is a fact to a certain degree. But, only as much

time as you take to prepare your juice or protein shakes. In fact, most of the time there is very little cooking time involved. You can prepare and carry such diets easily. There is no fuss about heating or freezing as most of the items are fresh.

The preparation time for an anti-inflammatory diet is also similar to the time taken for preparing a regular meal. Of course, it will be higher as compared to the processed food, but then you are eating away the chances of a healthy life then.

A healthy diet is the biggest gift you can give to yourself. It plays a decisive role in your health. It deserves a little bit of your time, and it isn't demanding much from you. There are scores of recipes to prepare tasty salads, breakfasts, lunches, and dinners. Some preparations change like frying gets replaced by baking and grilling.

Limited Food Choices

If you are considering anti-inflammatory diet, then I believe this is an incorrect question to consider. Inflammation naturally limits the products you can consume. However, within the permitted and healthy food items, you have complete liberty to experiment. People generally consider the Mediterranean cuisine to be the ideal one. It has its natural advantages as it lays great stress on salads and light foods. Yet, there are numerous spices you can add to your food to make it tasty. Ginger, garlic, chili, turmeric, cumin, cinnamon and scores of others to choose from. The taste will have a new meaning for you. In place of adding lots of saturated fat, you can grill your food and dress it with healthy options like olive oil. The taste of the food will come out excellently. This doesn't have a fear of inflammations and no guilt trips either.

It is a choice you'll make.; the choice towards a healthy life. The limitations are just in our brain only until the time we take the initiative. This diet can give you a new lease of life if you are suffering from any of the earlier discussed problems. This diet will rejuvenate you and make you feel fresh, lively and energetic.

Anti-inflammatory diet along with physical activity can work wonders. Both have anti-inflammatory properties and work as antioxidants. The combo will not only help you in managing your stress levels but will also improve your sleep quality.

Chapter 5
The Ways to Make Your Anti-Inflammatory Diet Awesome

The biggest concern people have with adopting an anti-inflammatory diet is that it will be bland and tasteless. This is largely a misconception. An anti-inflammatory diet does advise you to cut down your salt, sugar and saturated fat usage, but it doesn't mean it takes away the taste. You can add taste by using natural sweeteners, spices, yogurt, and other healthy variants. A healthy anti-inflammatory diet apart from all the ingredients is also all about a positive attitude. You will certainly have to make some positive changes to your diet, but that is all for your health. Every time you eat something bad you have to bear the pain the next day in a form of digestion problems or inflammation in any other area. Such foods can also lead to chronic illnesses that can make you very sick. An anti-inflammatory diet will reduce the risk of chronic illnesses, and you wouldn't have digestive issues or unnecessary inflammations the next day. You wouldn't need to think before eating, a great shift from the current dilemma. You will have to make up your mind for once and get set on the path to good health. You can add taste, sweetness and other flavors to your food through natural alternatives given below.

Add herbs and spices to your diet

All the good things in life aren't tasteless, and spices are a live testimony of this fact. Spices are aromatic, healthy and make your food delicious. Spices like cinnamon, clove, cardamom, and black pepper have strong anti-inflammatory properties. They are full of antioxidants and help you in fighting various infections. They aid digestion and power your system to fight chronic illnesses. The health benefits of these spices are numerous. But when it comes to taste, they work wonderfully. They add aroma and taste to your food. They can make any food interesting by the smell and flavor. You can sprinkle them on your salads and use them lavishly in your curries as per your taste. They will make your soups tempting and crave for more.

One of the biggest advantages of spices is that they aid in digestion. The better your digestive system process the food you eat, the lower the chances of inflammation will be. Spices are very helpful, and they release a lot of antioxidants that fight the free radicals. This has been among the prime reasons they have been priced so high since the beginning of the trade. You can easily get them at grocery stores, and there are no chances that you can go wrong with spices. The best thing is that there is no health capping on the use of spices. You can use as many healthy spices as per your taste. Experiment with them and adjust them as per your taste your taste buds and make your food tasty and flavorful.

Use natural sweeteners like fruits, fruit juice, and honey

Craving for sweets is a natural tendency. Anyone can have a sweet tooth, but this gives way to a lot of troubles. Refined sugar not only increases the fructose levels, but it also gives birth to several issues like insulin resistance and obesity. The easy, simple and healthy way to fulfill your needs to have sugar is to rely on natural sweets like fruits, fruit juice, and honey.

You can eat fruits raw or even use them in your preparations to get natural sweet flavors. Nature has created a lot of varieties by making sweet fruits vary in taste. Some are sweet while some have a tangy taste. You can use them as per your liking. Fruit juices are very healthy, and you can also use them in your food preparations. Fruit juice, when used in meat recipes, tenderizes them and prevents the formation of harmful chemicals.

Honey has been used for thousands of years and has a strong anti-inflammatory effect. It is a great dietary supplement and natural sweetener. It is a healing agent and works magic on your digestive system. You can use honey in most of your recipes, and you'll never think of sugar once you understand the immense health benefits offered by honey.

Yogurt can enrich the flavors

Yogurt is healthy and tasty. You can use it in your smoothies and recipes. It is affordable and has a very good impact on your digestive system. The health benefits of yogurt are numerous. It helps your immune system, keeps your blood pressure in control, and reduces bad cholesterol apart from other advantages. You can make it a part of your diet and make your anti-inflammatory diet rich, healthy and tasty.

Chapter 6
Food Items to Include In Your Anti-Inflammatory Diet

Fruits

Fruits are the nature's gift to the mankind. They have a natural sweetness. Some have exotic taste, and others are full of nutrition. The main thing is that you can't go wrong with a fruit-filled diet in your anti-inflammatory diet.

Fruits are extremely rich in carotenoids and flavonoids. They are powerful antioxidants and boost anti-inflammatory activity. You will have a wide variety of fruits to choose from. The trick is to go for fresh organic fruits.

The red pulp fruits like cherries, strawberries, raspberries, blueberries, and blackberries are rich in anthocyanins. It has a strong anti-inflammatory effect.

Citrus fruits like orange, grapefruits, and lime are also rich in vitamin C. It can help in preventing inflammatory arthritis.

Fruits come in the top list of food items to be consumed in the highest quantity. They have specific advantages. They do not need to be cooked. They are highly nutritious and flavorful. They boost immunity and taste to your life. They are a ready meal. You can eat them on the go. Replacing the urge to gorge fast food with fruits is the healthiest alternative.

Some of the most beneficial anti-inflammatory fruits are:

Berries

Berries are small wonder fruits. They are luscious, tempting and mouthwatering. If anyone believes that all the good things in this world are bad in taste, he or she should reconsider while talking about berries. They are so delightful that you'll surely look for more. But, the taste is not the only gift. Berries can tackle chronic inflammation to a great extent. Berries are packed with inflammation-fighting antioxidants. Berries like blackberries, blueberries, cranberries, red raspberries, and strawberries have a great impact on the markers inducing chronic inflammations such as cancer, heart diseases, diabetes, and age-related mental disorders.

You can eat them as it is or also make lip-smacking smoothies. The sugar content of the berries is very helpful and will provide you the sugar punch you badly need. They are full of fiber, minerals, vitamins, and anthocyanins.

Apricots

This golden fruit comes with the first breeze of summers. It is full of vitamin C and A and has plenty of beta-carotene and fiber. Apricots are also very rich in antioxidants like flavonoids. Its health benefits are immense, and one of the most distinguishing quality is the ability to reduce the risk of heart diseases. Catechin an active phytonutrient present in apricots that inhibits the functioning of an enzyme called cyclooxygenase-2 (COX-2). COX-2 is an inflammation-causing enzyme. If you are troubled by blood pressure related problems, apricots can definitely help you. It stops the inflammation in the blood vessels and also the subsequent damages.

This fiber-rich fruit also helps your digestive system and prevents inflammation in the gut. The soluble fiber in apricots is especially very effective in controlling blood cholesterol levels.

Apricots are easily available across the US and have a fairly long season. They can be used in several delicious recipes to make your meals nutritious and tasty.

Cantaloupe

If oxidative stress is the cause of your inflammation and you need a blast of antioxidants, phytonutrients, and electrolytes, then this golden orange pulpy fruit has the magic potion for you. It is an effective answer to most of the modern-day inflammation caused by diseases.

This fruit especially is effective for the patients suffering from neurodegenerative disorders. Parkinson's disease and Alzheimer patients can push off their condition better. It has two powerful antioxidants called carotenoids and cucurbitacin. These help in preventing the progress of inflammation causing these diseases as well as cancer and heart issues.

High dosage of vitamin C and A in the fruit also

helps in maintaining healthy mucous membrane and promotes cellular health. The seeds of this fruit are a very rich source of omega-3 fatty acids.

Intake of this fruits leads to reduced levels of C reactive protein in the bloodstream. It is important to note here that C reactive protein works as a marker of inflammation. The dangers of chronic inflammation and autoimmune disorder decrease to a great extent with the use of this fruit.

It also helps in many heart-related problems like high cholesterol, and high blood pressure by reducing the oxidative stress.

You can make smoothies from it, use it as a salad or make jam, soup or sorbet. It tastes delicious in all the ways.

Peach

Peach is a fruit that has magical anti-inflammatory and anti-fungal properties. It works like a charm on free radicals and is full of antioxidants. Peach helps in preventing several cancers, heart diseases and keeps your gut healthy.

Peach is rich in antioxidants. It helps in keeping the free radicals in check. Its skin, pulp, and seed have strong properties that help in combating cancer. A unique combination of bioactive compounds in this fruit considerably reduce the risk of heart diseases in the users. It suppresses the production of inflammatory cytokines and histamines in the bloodstream that cause allergic reactions and inflammation. It is a golden fruit for the people with a sensitive gut. Its pulp not only helps in treating certain cancers but also provides relief in gut problems like motility disorder. It also has strong anti-fungal properties too. Its use can eliminate the growth of candida fungus in the users.

Peach shake will provide you lots of vitamin A, C and K, and magnesium. You can make great salads and desserts using peach or enjoy it in the natural form. Whatever way you use it, you are bound to get lots of nutrition and antioxidants.

Plum

This is a fleshy fruit surrounding a single hard seed. Eating dried plums on an empty stomach will make you feel fuller. It works great for controlling obesity and reducing the risk of diabetes and heart diseases. It is full of vitamin C and phytonutrients that help in preventing cell damage. They are full of dietary fiber and work wonders in regulating the digestive system. People suffering from chronic constipation will love it. It has a lot of soluble fibers that lowers the bad cholesterol in the bloodstream.

Out of some specific advantages of this fruit, one is its rich composition of phytonutrients. It helps in slowing down the inflammation in neurological areas. If a person is suffering from a neurological degenerative disorder like Alzheimer's or Parkinson's disease, then this fruit can provide great help. Vitamin C in the fruit is great for boosting immunity and reducing inflammation. This sweet fruit has a very low glycemic index. This means that you can lower your blood glucose levels by eating it.

Plum is a great breakfast fruit. You can eat this soft, sweet and easy to digest fruit in its natural form or use it in a pancake recipe. You can also add it to your smoothies or use it in various salads. Whichever way you use it, the anti-inflammatory effect remains great.

Grapefruit

It is a wonder fruit for the calorie conscious ones. It is significantly low in calories but high in vitamin C content. This citrus fruit has many important agents like lycopene and beta-carotene, limonoids and flavonoids. They boost immunity, accelerate weight loss and enhance metabolism. The users will get great assistance from within for losing weight. The fruit energizes the metabolic system which makes you energetic. The vitamin C and phytonutrients like limonin reduce the risk of various cancers. The high amount of flavonoid present in the fruit will significantly reduce the risk of strokes. It boosts your immune system and brings a glow to your skin. It stands very low on the glycemic index and hence if you are avoiding sugar, then this makes your life sweeter without causing any harm. In fact, it will lower the blood glucose levels in your bloodstream.

The best way to enjoy this delicious fruit is to make its juice or a smoothie. The refreshing taste of this fruit will revitalize your senses.

Kiwi

Kiwi is a power fruit. Even a small kiwi is oozing with vitamin C, E, and antioxidants. It has a great mix of phytonutrients, vitamins, and minerals. This citrus fruit can fulfill your complete need of vitamin C.

Kiwi gives you a high dosage of antioxidants that boost your immune system. It aids your digestive system and soothes your gut. It also has amazing antibacterial and antimicrobial capabilities. It reduces the risk of heart diseases by keeping the blood pressure in check.

Apart from other anti-inflammatory qualities, Kiwi

works especially well in improving your skin health. It has anti-aging properties. The serotonin content in the fruit has sleep aiding qualities. It improves the quality of your sleep and even helps you in coming out of mood swings and depression.

You can eat Kiwi fruit raw or even use it in baked items. You can also make its juice. Kiwi smoothies as especially liked by most.

Lemons and limes

Lemons and limes add flavor to our lives. These citrus fruits are loaded with antioxidants and vitamin C.

They make up a perfect anti-inflammatory food as they are low in calories but high in fiber and minerals. Lemon and lime can boost your immunity and ease up on inflammation. If you are at a high risk of heart diseases, then they will prove to be a treat for you. The antioxidants in them reduce the risk of heart diseases.

The best impact of lemons and limes has been studied on various types of cancers. The constituents of lime juice inhibit the growth of many types of cancer cells. You can also use lemon juice for preventing kidney stones. If you are susceptible to stones, then adding limes and lemons to your daily diet is a prudent idea. Additionally, lemon juice also provides great help in weight loss. It has low calories and high-fiber content that promotes weight loss.

You can make detox drinks from lemon juice or use it to garnish your salads. Lemon juice mixed with other herbs like thyme and rosemary constitutes a very healthy and flavorful combo.

Papaya

Papaya is a tropical detoxifying fruit. It has excellent anti-inflammatory properties and works wonders to aid digestion. Papaya is full of vitamins, minerals, flavonoids, and antioxidants that encourage great health.

Papaya is a magical fruit for many inflammatory conditions like leaky gut, inflammatory bowel syndrome, constipation, arthritis, asthma, heart diseases, certain cancers and macular degeneration.

A specific compound by the name of papain found in papaya has great ability to break apart the bond between amino acids. This provides great assistance in the digestion of complex foods like meat. It has excellent anti-inflammatory properties. It can provide great relief from diseases like asthma and arthritis.

The antioxidant properties of papaya help in curbing the free radical. It inhibits cholesterol from forming plaques along the artery walls. Papaya also decreases the risk of some types of cancers to a great extent. If age-related vision issues have been troubling you recently then also papaya is a great fruit for you. The flavonoids present in the fruit help in slowing macular degeneration and help you in maintaining good vision.

Papaya also has antiviral properties too. It can help you in fighting several viral infections. Papaya is a delicious fruit with several uses. It is a sweet fruit. You can use it to make juice, salads, salsa or desserts.

Pineapple

Pineapple is a sweet and tangy nutrient-dense fruit.

This tropical fruit is low in calories but very high in vitamin C, B1, potassium, manganese, antioxidants, and phytonutrients. It is a natural remedy to many problems ranging from issues like indigestion to allergies. Pineapple is a great home remedy if you frequently get a cough, cold or flu. It strengthens your immune system and protects you from such problems. It works like a charm in skin problems. High quantity of vitamin C in the fruit helps you in healing skin disorders. The fruit also has a very high ratio of fiber content. It is excellent for digestion. It lowers the risk of colorectal cancer significantly.

Pineapple is a great fruit for diabetic people. It not only gives them the required dosage of sweeteners but also lowers blood glucose levels. The high quality of antioxidants present in the fruit help in reducing the damage to the heart caused by the free radicals.

If you are allergic to certain things or foods or have asthma then also pineapple is a gift for you. The beta-carotene present in the fruit lowers their risk. Apart from these, pineapple is also good for mental upliftment. It can help in getting over depression and anxiety issues.

Its contribution to the digestive tract is also commendable. It can help in curing acid refluxes. It also eases the symptoms of gut inflammation and assists the digestive process. You can also use pineapple for joint pain and arthritis. It helps in relieving the pain.

Pineapple is a delicious fruit. Ripe pineapple can be eaten. It can also be used for making delicious juice, shake, smoothies and other drinks. It is widely used in several food preparations and desserts too. Pineapple makes an excellent salad ingredient. You can enjoy it the way you like and get the benefits of natural remedy.

Banana

Banana is a portable, affordable and low in calorie fruit. It is full of sugar that's good for our health. Bananas provide lots of carbohydrates in the form of quick releasing sugar. If you need quick energy after a workout or you're feeling hungry then grabbing a banana is the best choice. Bananas are also a rich source of potassium.

They help in managing your blood flow and provide assistance in managing your blood pressure. They can help in decreasing the symptoms of kidney stones, gout, ADHD, back pain, and headache.

Banana has a lot of fiber. This helps you in digestion and is an excellent remedy for constipation, bloating and other digestive problems. Bananas also help in preventing many mood disorders like anxiety and depression. Bananas contain manganese that is very important for maintaining a healthy brain function. It is a very useful remedy for disorders like epilepsy and Parkinson's disease. Bananas have several anti-inflammatory properties as well as have ample antioxidants. It is a food that can become an important part of your anti-inflammatory diet.

You can eat bananas as a fruit. You can also use them in salads, or make delicious smoothies and shakes. You can put them in pancakes, muffins, and bread to make interesting recipes.

Vegetables

Vegetables are a rich source of flavonoids and carotenoids, and they boost immunity and reduce oxidative stress. An anti-inflammatory diet without green leafy vegetables and cruciferous vegetables will be incomplete. You can eat many vegetables raw or cooked. They provide you the required nutrients and help in fighting inflammation. Vegetables are a very affordable source of nutrition, and they add taste to your plate. There is a wide variety of vegetables to choose from, and you can never get bored. The bright colored veggies are not only a treat for your taste buds but, they are a feast for eyes too.

The anti-inflammatory properties of vegetables are very high, and that's why they stand at the top of the chain. The only thing to remember is giving the right treatment and choosing the correct vegetables as per your needs. The following list will tell you the best vegetables to be included in your list and the amazing nutritional and anti-inflammatory properties they possess.

Spinach

Spinach is a superfood. It is a nutrient-dense food that can fulfill a lot of your nutritional needs. Spinach is filled with a dozen of flavonoids that act as antioxidants and have amazing anti-inflammatory properties. It has a very positive impact on your central nervous system and reduces inflammation. If you are concerned about the accelerated signs of aging, then it is a wonder food for you. It can delay signs of aging and bring amazing glow.

One of the best qualities about spinach is that it has protective carotenoids that significantly decrease the risk of many diseases like cancer, heart problems, diabetes, neurodegenerative disorders like Alzheimer's and Parkinson's disease and obesity.

The antioxidant-rich spinach helps in fighting free radicals. This is very important for remaining safe from inflammation and heart diseases. It is also a rich source of Vitamin C and A. You will have a strong immune system and wonderful eyesight. Spinach provides you ample amount of minerals such as manganese, zinc, and selenium that help in maintaining an excellent digestive system.

Cancer is a big risk in the current times, and spinach is a superfood for decreasing the risk of cancer. Several studies have proven that it can slow down the cancerous cell formation. It limits the inflammation in the body to a great extent limiting the development risk factors associated with heart diseases and blood pressure. This fiber-rich food also helps in lowering your cholesterol levels and slows down the absorption of glucose in the bloodstream. The antioxidants in spinach can reduce the oxidative stress that might lead to a decline in cognitive, behavioral and motor skills.

You can boil, sauté, steam, or bake spinach for preparing tasty recipes or even eat it raw and fresh. It is a great ingredient for salads and smoothies. It is one of the healthiest foods available to mankind and will make a great addition to your anti-inflammatory diet.

Broccoli

Broccoli is loaded with oxidants that help in fighting cancer. It is full of fiber and other vitamins and minerals. It is one of the most valuable foods. It promotes good health and longevity. No other food items beat it when it comes to preventing cancer. It is full of antioxidants and enzymes that help in slowing down the death of cells and cell cycles. It is a rich source of isothiocyanates which is phytonutrient that stimulates detoxifying enzymes. It is also a good source of vitamin B6 that stimulates brain health. It works very well in lowering the cholesterol levels and high blood pressure.

High levels of vitamin A in Broccoli promote skin and eye health. Broccoli is also a good source of vitamin K, calcium and potassium. They help in maintaining healthy bones, nails, and teeth. The high fiber content in broccoli is good for your digestive tract. It prevents constipation, IBS, and other digestive issues. The anti-inflammatory properties of broccoli are very strong, and it is a magic food for people looking for good health. It detoxifies your body and strengthens your immunity. It is an excellent food for encouraging hormonal health. If you are conscious about your weight management then also broccoli is a great vegetable for you. It ensures better cognitive functions even in advancing age.

Broccoli is a vegetable that goes well with varied flavors and cuisines. You can eat it in your breakfast, lunch and dinner alike. A combination of broccoli with other vegetables like tomato, onion, garlic, ginger, parsley, lemon will increase the taste. You can have it as a salad ingredient and eat it raw, boiled or roasted. Whatever the way you choose keeping it as an essential part of your diet will take you a long way ahead on the path to good health. It is a great vegetable to be included in the anti-inflammatory diet.

Celery

Celery is an excellent source of antioxidants and beneficial enzymes. It is also rich in vitamin K, C, and B6 along with minerals like potassium and folate. Celery is a vegetable that has proven effective in reducing high blood pressure, high cholesterol. It is a gift for your heart as it has a lot of antioxidants. However, the benefits just don't end here, it is also a rich source of dietary fiber. It gives a great boost to your digestive system and also promotes weight loss. So, all the people aiming to reduce weight must take a note of that.

The flavonoids and phytonutrients present in celery also help in improving cognitive health. You can eat the stalk, leaves, and seeds of celery and everything will be beneficial. It is a minimal waste vegetable. The anti-inflammatory properties of celery reduce the oxidative stress and fight the free radicals in your body. It is very effective in many chronic inflammations causing cancer, heart diseases, and arthritis. The anti-microbial properties of celery help in fighting infections. It is also very effective in curing bacterial infections of the digestive tract. So, if you regularly suffer from urinary tract infections, bladder disorders, kidney problems and cysts, then celery will be a great addition to your anti-inflammatory diet.

It is best not to overcook celery as that will destroy the useful antioxidants in it. Steaming it keeps most of the nutrients intact. You can eat it in salads, stir-fry it other vegetables or make delicious and healthy smoothies and juices along with other vegetables. You can also eat it raw. It always works best as a garnishing material. Always go for organic celery as that is the best and free from harmful spray of pesticides.

Turnip Greens

Turnip greens like all other green leafy vegetables are a rich source of vitamins, minerals, and antioxidants. They are a good candidate to be included in your anti-inflammatory diet. It is a leafy vegetable with amazing ability to fight chronic inflammations like cancers and heart diseases. It gives a great boost to your detox system, immunity and liver function. It lowers the free radical damage and reduces inflammations that may lead to chronic diseases to a great extent. It is very good for people with higher risk of diabetes, arthritis, autoimmune disorders, Alzheimer's and Parkinson's disease. It slows down the cognitive decline and promotes better brain function.

You can enjoy the benefits of turnip greens by quickly boiling them for a short while and then refreshing them in cold water. You can also sauté them. This green leafy vegetable is filled with nutrients and antioxidants that make it a great addition to an anti-inflammatory diet.

Zucchini

Zucchini forms a low carb diet with the very low score on the glycemic index. It is an ideal vegetable for the weight conscious people. The high percentage of water in zucchini makes it low in calories, carbs, and sugar but high in essential nutrients like potassium, manganese, vitamin C and vitamin A.

Zucchini works very well in lowering blood pressure, fighting against inflammation, and clearing clogged arteries. It boosts your immune system and has antimicrobial and antiparasitic properties. It has several beneficial effects on your gut, nervous, immune and cardiovascular system. The raw seeds of zucchini are helpful in providing protein nutrition, reducing free radical damage and oxidation. It has amazing anti-inflammatory properties that boost your heart health. It lowers the harmful cholesterol levels and improves the health of the arteries by reducing the risk of diseases causing inflammation.

This low sugar and low carb diet can support your weight loss efforts. It is also very good for your digestive system and helps in reducing IBS, ulcer symptoms and leaky gut syndrome. It is also very good for people suffering from thyroid, and insulin regulation issues.

You can eat it raw, cook or even grill it. It cooks pretty quickly and consumes the least amount of time.

Brussels Sprouts

Brussels sprouts are crunchy, versatile and delicious. Their nutritional value is immense as they are loaded with antioxidants and help in fighting cancer and heart diseases. They are full of vitamin K, vitamin A, vitamin B, vitamin C, potassium, manganese and other nutrients. They also help you in minimizing the risk of obesity, diabetes and neurodegenerative disorders along with bigger issues like cancer and heart diseases.

The antioxidants and phytonutrients in the brussels sprouts lower the risk of cancer and heart diseases by reducing the free radical damage. They also provide you with vitamin K which is the bone building material. It also helps you in curing digestive and intestinal problems. Rich in vitamin C it helps in reducing inflammation and cell damage. The potassium in Brussels sprout also helps in proper nerve function and improves brain health.

You can get the most out of brussels sprouts by

roasting or sautéing them. Overcooking them might take away most of the nutrients. Steaming is also a good way to enjoy this vegetable.

Carrot

Carrot is a highly effective anti-inflammatory vegetable that tastes good and can be eaten raw, cooked or juiced. Full of carotenoids, carrots play an important role in fighting free radical damage. If you are at a high risk of cancer or heart diseases, then carrots are an ideal vegetable to be included in your anti-inflammatory diet. Carrots provide ample amounts of vitamin C, D, E and K along with minerals like magnesium, potassium, and calcium. The high fiber content in carrots gives a boost to your digestive system.

Carrots facilitate faster wound healing and have a very positive impact on your brain health and cognitive functions.

You can enjoy carrots any way you like. Eat them raw, and in salads, they are a great addition to any salad. You can cook them and make delicious soups and stews. Carrot juice needs no introduction at all. It provides concentrated nutrition and has amazing health benefits.

Asparagus

Asparagus has gained the status of being one of the fanciest selling vegetables. This nutrient-dense vegetable is a rich source of folic acid, potassium, fiber, vitamin B6, A, C, K, and thiamine. Asparagus works best in reducing the effect of cell-damaging free radicals. It is packed with anti-inflammatory properties and antioxidants which even gives it a medicinal effect. This low-calorie food contains no fat at all while being loaded with vitamins and minerals.

Asparagus has strong anti-inflammatory properties, and it is full of antioxidants that help in reducing the risk of chronic illnesses like type 2 diabetes, heart diseases, and cancer. It also has a great anti-aging effect. The diuretic properties of asparagus also aid in the production of urine. This is especially helpful for people with high blood pressure and urinary tract infections.

One of the most striking qualities of asparagus is the inulin content. It is a nutrient that passes undigested to our large intestine and becomes the food of good bacteria. This particularly helps in lowering the risk of allergies and colon cancer.

The thiamine in asparagus helps in improving the cellular function. The detoxifying compounds in asparagus help in help in reduction of carcinogens in our body. It lowers the risk of many types of cancers.

You can roast it, microwave it or grill it to your heart's content. Garnish it with spices to make a healthy meal or eat it like an appetizer. Adding it to your anti-inflammatory diet will be a very wise decision.

Cauliflower

Cauliflower is one of the most prominent members of the cruciferous vegetable family. Full of phytonutrients and antioxidants this vegetable brings a number of health benefits with it. Cauliflower helps in preventing a large number of chronic illnesses like heart diseases, diabetes, many types of cancers and neurodegenerative disorders. It is full of antioxidants, minerals and vitamins C and K. It detoxifies your body and helps in losing weight.

If you are troubled with imbalanced hormones then also cauliflower is a great vegetable for your diet.

The anti-inflammatory qualities of cauliflower are huge. The omega-3 fatty acids in cauliflowers help in keeping the arteries and blood vessels free from plaque.

Cauliflower is easy to prepare and tastes amazing. You can grill, boil, stir-fry, or microwave as you like.

Onion

Onion is a strong candidate in the anti-inflammatory list that only provides a lot of antioxidants but also tastes to your meals. It has a lot of flavonoids and polyphenols that are good for your blood sugar level, bones, and inflammation.

Onion is a vegetable that increases the taste of any meal and makes a great addition to your salads. It is flavor rich and full of health benefits. It works great in reducing the risk of various diseases like arthritis, diabetes, asthma and neurodegenerative disorders. It is full of therapeutic oils that are especially helpful in fighting cancer-causing cells.

List of anti-inflammatory benefits of onions is long, and it will suffice to say that this vegetable will keep many diseases at bay. They carry the lowest risk of pesticide contamination as their natural structure doesn't allow it. You can mix them with many vegetables and prepare side dishes or main course.

Cucumber

Cucumber has many positive things to cite under its belt, but its most striking quality is to act like a free radical scavenger. It works like your personal free radical policing system which either stops them from propping up or eliminates them before they cause any damage. It is full of antioxidants like flavonoids and tannins and has amazing cancer-fighting abilities. It can minimize the oxidative stress and reduce the risk of various tumors.

Cucumber has very high fiber and water content which makes a darling of weight conscious people. It cleans your liver and detoxifies your body. It is excellent for your digestion and helps in constipation. It works great as an anti-inflammatory vegetable. You can eat it raw, use it in salads or juice it. The crunchy, watery flavor of cucumber is heavenly. Cooking them doesn't produce a very good result as it can become limp. You can pickle it to get different flavors.

Sweet Potato

Sweet potato is an interesting choice for an anti-inflammatory diet. Both parts of its name sweet and potato are enough for raising many eyebrows. Yet, they can prove you wrong every time.

Sweet potatoes have anti-diabetic properties, and they help in regulating your blood sugar levels. They also help in improving your insulin sensitivity. Although they have potato in their name yet, they no contribute towards weight gain. On the contrary, they are nutrient dense and stuffed with fiber. This helps in improving your digestive system and making you feel fuller faster. You will be able to lose weight faster if you have sweet potatoes in your diet. Sweet potatoes are rich in antioxidants that lead to the elimination of free radicals. They reduce the risk of diabetes, heart diseases, and cancers. Sweet potatoes also help in boosting brain function and improve memory. Your immunity will increase by making them a part of your diet plan.

You can microwave, bake, boil, grill, sauté or roast sweet potatoes and they'll taste delicious.

Whole Grains

Whole grains are essential for you. They supply the essential fibers that are a must for your digestive system health. They take time to get digested, and this slow process reduces the chances of a spike in blood sugar levels and inflammation. They have several other nutrients too apart from high fiber content that is essential for you. Missing out on whole grains will not be a very wise decision for you. You can make a variety of dishes from whole grains, and they'll make you feel fuller pretty faster. This will also help in your weight loss efforts.

Quinoa

Quinoa has gained good recognition in the past some time, and there is a great ground for that. It is one of the best complete protein food available, and it is gluten-free. It has several advantages that keep it ahead of other food items, yet the presence of high amounts of disease-fighting antioxidants take the cake. It has strong anti-inflammatory properties and will work great for you. It is gluten-free and aids your weight loss efforts too. Quinoa is very good for your heart, and it also helps you in fighting cancer.

Quinoa is also very good for your digestive system as it contains indigestible fiber. This is especially beneficial for the growth of the good bacteria in your gut. High manganese, magnesium and phosphorus content in quinoa support bone health and also reduce the risk of diabetes.

There is a lot you can do with quinoa. You can make

quinoa flour or use it as a pilaf or even make porridge. All you need to do is pick it up from any grocery store and try to use as per your liking.

Barley

Barley is a great candidate for this list as it is a high fiber whole grain. It is also full of vitamins, minerals, and antioxidants apart from the fiber. Barley is one of the best grain for improving your gut health. The high fiber content keeps your digestive tract healthy. It also aids your weight loss efforts as you feel fuller faster with barley. Barley helps in managing your blood sugar levels as it slows down the release of sugar into the bloodstream. The propionic acid in barley inhibits the production of enzymes that lead to the production of cholesterol. This lowers your cholesterol levels and keeps your heart healthy. It also has phytonutrients that help in fighting chronic inflammation. It also has a large number of vitamins and minerals that aid your overall health. In all, barley is a very healthy grain to be included in an anti-inflammatory diet.

Buckwheat

Buckwheat is a superfood. It is a nutrient dense and gluten-free seed that is full of inflammation-fighting antioxidants. Buckwheat is protein and fiber. It is very good for your digestive system and prevents diseases like diabetes and heart problems. It has many antioxidants like rutin, tannins, catechin that help in fighting illnesses. One of the best things about buckwheat is that it doesn't contain gluten. It is non-allergic, and you can consume it without fear of allergic symptoms.

Buckwheat is rich in many vital nutrients like vitamins and minerals that are essential for a healthy body. It makes your food complete and wholesome. It provides you highly digestible proteins that are usually absent in plant-based nutrition.

You can use buckwheat as a healthy side dish in place of rice or use it to make porridge. You can use it to make pancakes and also use it in addition to soups and stews.

Oats

There's very little need to talk about the benefits of oats as they are quite popular. The health benefits of eating oats are many, but the best thing about oats is that they are easy to prepare.

Oats are very good for your heart as they help in lowering your cholesterol levels. They have a high percentage of belly-filling fiber that makes you fuller faster, and hence they support weight loss. They aid your digestion and provide relief from problems like constipation.

Oats are a great addition to your anti-inflammatory diet as they contain polysaccharides that help in enhancing immune function. They have a low glycemic score and are a rich source of manganese and phosphorus.

There are scores of recipes that can be prepared with oats and they are fairly easy to cook.

Brown Rice

Brown rice is a gluten-free food. It is loaded with vitamins, minerals, fiber, and protein. It can reduce the risk of problems like diabetes and heart diseases. Brown rice is rich in magnesium that helps your heart. It is also a rich source of manganese that aids the production of digestive enzymes. It also decreases your bad cholesterol levels and boosts your immune system. It is a low-calorie food, and hence you can eat it without the fear of gaining excess weight.

Rye

Rye is among the healthiest grains. The health benefits of rye are immense, and you can't go wrong by keeping rye in your anti-inflammatory diet. It helps you fight several problems like heart diseases, diabetes, chronic inflammation, high blood pressure and even cancer. It helps in weight loss too.

Rye is a cholesterol-lowering food, and it improves your insulin sensitivity. It effectively helps in weight management too. Rye has excellent anti-inflammatory properties, and it helps in improving your immune system. It has several phytonutrients that help in fighting cancer.

One important thing to remember is that it isn't gluten free although its gluten content is lower than wheat flour. So if you have gluten intolerance, then you might want to avoid it.

Beans and Legumes

Beans and legumes are a very rich source of protein. They provide you a high amount of fiber that helps you in managing your digestive system and also regulate your blood sugar levels. They are very good at managing bad cholesterol and help you in flushing out the toxins from your body.

Keeping them in your anti-inflammatory diet will not only add variety to your diet, but it will also bring several health benefits too. You can create variations as per your taste and enjoy the benefits of good health. Keeping them in the diet is very important especially for the vegetarian people as beans and legumes fulfill the protein needs.

Black Beans

Black beans are an affordable source of protein, fiber, vitamins, minerals, and antioxidants. They can prevent chronic inflammation, heart diseases, diabetes and some type of cancers too. Black beans have several phytonutrients that help in fighting long-term inflammation. It also helps in improving your cardiovascular health. There are several antioxidants in the black beans that help in fighting many types of cancers. They fight free radical damage and reduce the oxidative stress.

The thing that makes black beans in addition to a regular diet is the fact that they are exceptionally rich in fiber. They improve your digestive health and clean your body of toxic chemicals. They are very low on the glycemic index and hence keep your blood sugar levels stable.

Black beans contain several essential vitamins and minerals like folate, copper, magnesium, phosphorus and B vitamins. They help you in maintaining a healthy body.

Lentils

Lentils are very high in protein. They help in improving your heart function, regulate your blood sugar level and improve your digestive health. Lentils have a high amount of filling fiber. This fiber helps in several ways like it makes you feel fuller faster. It also absorbs the excess toxins and fat and carries it out of your body. The soluble fiber in the lentils lowers the cholesterol levels in your blood preventing heart diseases. Lentils balance the pH levels in your body and maintain a healthy gut environment.

They are a very good source of protein and hence if you are a vegetarian, then they can become your important source of protein. The dietary fiber in lentil also improves your immune system. It reduces the oxidative damage and flushes out the toxins from your body. They are a great addition to an anti-inflammatory diet.

Kidney Beans

Kidney beans are low in fat and rich in minerals, proteins, vitamins, and carbohydrates. They reduce the risk of heart diseases, diabetes, and cancer. They are packed with fiber and various other nutrients that make them ideal for reducing fat.

Kidney beans reduce the levels of bad cholesterol in your blood and decrease the risk of heart diseases. The high fiber content in kidney beans lowers the blood glucose and helps you in managing diabetes. They stand very low on the glycemic index and hence are very safe. They also have a higher percentage of flavonoids that help in fighting several types of cancers. If you are concerned about managing your weight then also these beans are very good for you. They have alpha-amylase inhibitors that help in managing weight. You must keep them in your anti-inflammatory diet.

Healthy Fats

Fat is also important. You cannot do away with fat content. But, it is important to consume only the good fats. Healthy fats are rich in omega-3 fatty acids or monosaturated fats. They give your body the ability to fight with free radical damage and have several antioxidants. You will need a healthy amount of these fats to reduce the oxidative stress and flavor your food. You can get these healthy fats from various sources apart from oils too. Fish are a rich source of omega-3 fatty acids. Nuts are also a rich source of healthy fats. You must have a balanced quantity of these fats to create a balance between the omega-6 fatty acids and omega-3 fatty acids in your body.

Extra Virgin Olive Oil

The whole world knows about extra virgin olive oils. They have uncountable benefits and provide you the essential monosaturated fats to you. Oleic acid one of the most common monosaturated fatty acid present in olive oil can fight free radical damage. It is extremely good for your heart. They reduce oxidative stress, inflammation, and microbial activity.

High level of antioxidants present in olive oil help in fighting inflammation. They are especially good for reducing the risk of cancer. Olive oil also helps your weight loss efforts as it controls excess insulin. It is good for your brain too as omega-3 fatty acids reduce the oxidative stress in the brain. The positive impact of olive oil on the skin is known globally.

Extra virgin olive oil is the best for your health. However, you can also use virgin olive oil. You need to buy these oils carefully as fake oils with a mix of other oils, or poorly processed oils are also available in plenty.

Avocado Oil

Avocado oil is one of the healthiest oils and has immense health benefits. It is especially beneficial for people with arthritis as it can reverse it. It can also help in preventing diabetes, high cholesterol, and obesity. Avocado oil is also known for curbing the high triglyceride levels. You can use it in salads, or cook with it as it has a very high smoke point.

The monosaturated fats in avocado oil help in maintaining healthy blood pressure. They are also helpful for various skin problems and psoriasis. The positive effect of avocado oil on the heart is also very high. The oleic acid in avocado oil helps in reducing the risk of heart diseases.

They have several antioxidants that help in fighting inflammation and aid nutrient absorption too.

Almonds

Almonds are known for their ability to reduce cholesterol levels. They have filling fiber, antioxidants, and plant protein. Almonds can reduce the risk of heart diseases considerably. They are rich in antioxidants that lower the risk of heart diseases and inflammation. They are also good for healthy brain function and prevent cognitive decline. The vitamin E content in almonds is very good for skin health. The monosaturated fatty acids in almonds help in managing blood sugar levels and prevent insulin resistance. They are good for your digestive system too as the fiber content in almonds is very high. The antioxidants present in almonds reduce the risk of oxidative stress leading to cancer.

Pistachio

Nutrient-dense pistachio is filled with healthy unsaturated fats. It helps you in weight loss and weight control and can be a very healthy snack item.

It lowers the bad cholesterol in your blood and boosts your eye health. It is very helpful for managing the risk of diabetes.

It is a tasty snack, and you can munch on it anytime. It has a very positive impact on your sexual function too.

Walnuts

Walnuts are the brain food. They can improve your mood and also help in fighting depression. Several studies have proven that walnuts are very good for preventing cognitive decline. Thus, regular consumption of walnuts can slow down age-related problems like dementia and Alzheimer's disease. They are rich in omega-3 fatty acids and help in fighting heart problems. They also help in lowering the triglyceride levels in your blood. The anti-inflammatory properties of walnuts also help in fighting the risk of several types of cancers.

Fish

Fish are a rich source of omega-3 fatty acids. They have strong anti-inflammatory properties and help in fighting chronic inflammation. Fish are an important part of an anti-inflammatory diet and enrich your food with taste and health benefits. However, you must choose the kinds of fish you eat. Wild caught cold water fishes are the best as they have the highest amount of omega-3 fatty acids. In case, you do not want to eat fish you can also include molecularly distilled fish oil supplements in your diet.

Salmon

Wild caught salmon is filled with vitamins, minerals, and omega-3 fatty acids. It is an important food item as it promotes whole body wellness. Apart from other health benefits, salmon has great ability to fight heart diseases and cancer. This omega-3 fatty acid rich food can increase brain efficiency and memory. It protects the nervous system from age-related damage and be used to treat Alzheimer's disease and Parkinson's symptoms. The anti-inflammatory properties of salmon help in preventing bone-related diseases and can help in keeping osteoporosis at away. Salmon also helps in defending your body against the onslaught of cancer and tumors. The omega-3 fatty acid content in the fish works excellently in preventing these diseases.

Sardines

Sardines are a great source of omega-3 fatty acids, vitamins, and minerals. They make a great anti-inflammatory food as the omega-3 fatty acid content reduces the risk of inflammations significantly. They improve your heart health and brain function too. They can help you in fighting a number of problems like mood disorders, anxiety, depression, arthritis, and cancers. They are full of essential vitamins and minerals like vitamin B12 and D along with calcium and selenium. They protect your bone health and also help in controlling blood sugar levels.

The risk of heart diseases also goes down with sardines due to the presence of omega-3 fatty acids. You can eat them for their taste and strong anti-inflammatory effect.

Herring

Herring is another fish that is good for your health. It is rich in omega-3 fatty acids, vitamin D, and minerals. It presents a strong defense against metabolic syndrome, heart diseases, and diabetes. It also reduces the risk of autoimmune disease syndrome to a large extent. If you are facing vitamin D deficiency, then herring is a good food choice for you due to its richness in vitamin D.

It also has a strong impact in lowering the risk of cognitive decline. It prevents memory loss and helps in curing depression. The high presence of omega-3 fatty acids in the fish is healthy for the heart and also helps in managing blood pressure. Its anti-inflammatory properties make it very suitable for fighting many types of cancers too.

Mackerel

Mackerel is an omega-3 powerhouse along with other micronutrients. Mackerels are nutrient dense with lots of omega-3 fatty acid and protein.

Among the main benefits of consuming mackerels are blood pressure and cholesterol management. They decrease the levels of triglycerides in your blood and protect your heart. High omega-3 fatty acid presence also ensures better brain function and helps in curing mood disorders. Mackerels also strengthen your bones and promote weight loss. Including them in your diet can be a very wise decision.

Spices and Herbs

Spices and herbs add flavor to your food and also to your life. They are healthy and have strong anti-inflammatory properties. Regular use of spices and herbs can protect you from many illnesses, and they can also negate the harmful effects of several food items you consume.

Spices and herbs are aromatic and bring color to your food. They make the food look and taste more appealing. You can add spices and herbs to your heart's content and as per your taste as there is no negative impact on your health. You should use them more often.

Turmeric

Turmeric is among the most miraculous herbs on this planet. It has strong anti-inflammatory properties and medicinal effects. It fights inflammation and stops many chronic illnesses from spreading. It is very effective for arthritis patients. Turmeric also slows down the formation of blood clots, and this reduces the risk of many clot-related problems. It is also found to be very effective in treating depression.

The effect of turmeric in diabetes and heart diseases is well known. It reduces the oxidative stress and activates the enzymes that lower the risk of diabetes. It is a natural pain reliever and detoxifies your body. Turmeric also has anticancer effects, and it can also help patients suffering from inflammatory bowel syndrome.

Ginger

Ginger has therapeutic and anti-inflammatory properties. Ginger has been in use around the world for its healing properties for centuries. High antioxidant and anti-inflammatory properties make it unique.

Ginger has powerful anti-fungal properties that make it very suitable to treat fungal infections. It is anti-bacterial and has also proven effective in treating bacterial infections.

Ginger also has anticancer properties that make it a great choice to be used for warding off the dangers of cancer. It can inhibit the synthesis of inflammation markers in the body reducing the risk of inflammation.

Ginger is also effective in controlling blood sugar levels and aids in digestion too.

Cinnamon

Cinnamon is a wonder spice. It has antioxidants, anti-inflammatory, ant-diabetic, and anti-microbial properties. It boosts your immunity and prevents chronic illnesses like diabetes, heart diseases, and cancer.

The high amount of antioxidants present in cinnamon prevent free radical damage and reduce the oxidative stress. It has strong anti-inflammatory properties that help in fighting dangerous infections. It reduces the cholesterol and triglyceride levels in your blood and gives relief in blood pressure and heart diseases. It is also very effective in slowing age-related cognitive degradation. People suffering from Alzheimer's disease and Parkinson's syndrome can especially benefit from the use of cinnamon.

The use of cinnamon strengthens your immune system and makes it capable of fighting various infections and viruses. It has anti-fungal, anti-bacterial and anti-microbial properties.

Chapter 7
The Plan to Get the Best from Your Anti-Inflammatory Diet

1. Fiber must be an essential part of your anti-inflammatory diet plan

Our digestive system plays a key role in our immune system. If the health of your digestive system is not good, then you will face chronic inflammations. Several diseases of the gut will occur, and there will be an imbalance between the good and bad bacteria that are present in the gut. Fiber helps in keeping your gut healthy. Dietary fiber is also important for maintaining a healthy blood glucose levels in your bloodstream. Fiber also increases the insulin sensitivity in your body. So, missing on a daily dose of at least 25g can prove to be a costly mistake.

Getting this much fiber is really easy. A good mix of fruits and vegetables along with whole grain will supply you more fiber than this. For instance, a single banana has 3 grams of fiber. It will help in reducing inflammation and fighting many chronic illnesses.

2. Fruits and Vegetables are your nutrient

supplements

All those people out there looking for the best nutrient supplements have all the reason to end their quest. Fruits and vegetables supply most of the nutrients required for a healthy body and mind. They are full of vitamins, minerals, and antioxidants. They are easy to digest and help in fighting inflammation.

Every day you must eat at least 4-5 servings of fruits and vegetables. Leafy greens, cruciferous and fruits are full of anti-inflammatory properties. Leaving them out can make your anti-inflammatory diet inefficient and ineffective. They add taste to your life and make you look healthy and energetic just like them.

3. Crucifers along with onion, ginger, and garlic can spell magic for your health

This is no secret that crucifers like broccoli, cauliflower, and brussels sprouts are full of nutrients. Their anti-inflammatory properties are very strong. You can increase their powers and taste many times by adding ginger, garlic, and onion to your preparations. They supplement each other and strengthen your immune system. Adding onion, ginger, and garlic will also give flavor to your dishes. You can also try adding other spices for taste.

4. Consuming more than 10 percent saturated fats can be counterproductive

High intake of saturated fats can spell trouble for you. They can increase the risk of heart diseases and lead to the release of free radicals. On a daily basis, you must not consume more than 20 grams of saturated fats per 2000 calorie intake.

You must reduce the consumption of red meat. It is difficult to digest and has a lot of fat. When you do eat it, marinate it with herbs, spices, vinegar and fresh fruit juices to reduce the build-up of toxic compounds during cooking.

5. Omega-3 fatty acids are very important

There are plenty of fruits, vegetables, seafood and nuts that provide omega-3 fatty acids. You must ensure that you are taking a good amount of those foods daily. Omega-3 fatty acids are very important for reducing inflammation and lowering the risk of diseases caused by chronic inflammation. Cancer, arthritis, heart diseases, neurodegenerative disorders are some of these diseases that can be prevented by including omega-3 fatty acids in your diet.

6. Include cold water fish in your diet more often

Wild cold water fishes like salmon, mackerel, trout are a very rich source of omega-3 fatty acids. They also provide most of the other essential vitamins and minerals. Eating wild caught cold water fish on a daily basis or at least few times a week will boost your immunity to a great extent. These fish provide all the necessary antioxidants that form an essential part of your anti-inflammatory diet. If you do not want to eat fish or face problems in getting wild caught cold water fish, you can also take molecularly distilled fish oil supplements. Missing out on either of the options will be really unfortunate.

7. Choose healthy oils for best results

Food may not look complete without oils and fat, yet being inconsiderate in the choice of oils can cost you a lot. Bad oil can cause a lot of damage to your heart and aid the production of free radicals. Although your body does need some fat, it doesn't need to be bad.

There are plenty of healthy options for oils like a virgin and extra virgin olive oil. You can also choose expeller pressed canola oil or sunflower oil. These are a rich source of polyphenols that act as antioxidants.

8. Use fruits and spices to make your meals delicious

It is very important to understand that all your hard work and self-control would go for a toss if you do not exercise self-control. Taste is an important part of life, and without it, things can get boring. Yet, looking for it in refined sugar and artificial sweeteners can be a big mistake. These products not only lead to excess accumulation of fructose but may also cause insulin resistance and increase the risk of type 2 diabetes.

Fruits are natural sweeteners. The sugar content in the fruits will help in regulating your blood sugar level, and the digestive fiber will absorb the extra glucose. You can keep your meals tasty while ensuring good health with fruits. Spices are another way of bringing flavor to meals. They not only increase the aroma and taste of your food but also make it very healthy. Spices like black pepper, cardamom, cloves, cinnamon, cumin, coriander and curry spices have strong anti-inflammatory properties. You will get better taste along with good health. They will supply the antioxidants and reduce the impact of the free radical damage.

9. 1 or 2 Servings per day of beans and legumes

will take you a long way

Most of the vegetables lose their nutrients if overcooked. However, it is not the case with beans and legumes. They can be cooked to heart's content and provide necessary minerals, protein, and soluble fiber. They are tasty and very healthy. Keeping them out of your daily dose of anti-inflammatory diet will create a deficiency.

10. Physical activity is also important

A very important fact that you must never forget is the importance of physical activity in your anti-inflammatory diet. Physical activity stimulates your immune system and helps your body in fighting inflammation. Your system will be able to absorb the required nutrients fast and fight better for chronic illnesses. Even small amounts of physical activity like a brisk walk can help in regulating your hormones and maintain a healthy balance. You will feel more refreshed and rejuvenated. It is one of the most important parts of an anti-inflammatory diet. You must understand that an anti-inflammatory diet is a holistic approach. It cannot be achieved through one-dimensional effort. You will have to put your mind, body, and soul to it.

Chapter 8
Foods to Avoid For a Healthy Body

An anti-inflammatory diet is all about making careful choices. You will have to choose dietary preferences that promote good health. You will also have to choose a healthy lifestyle that encourages better health. Leading a sedentary lifestyle might not help you in reaping the complete benefits of an anti-inflammatory diet.

However, the most important choice of all is to avoid the foods that cause inflammation. Causing any kind of damage is comparatively much easier task than repairing it. You must acknowledge this fact clearly. Even if you are eating the best food but do not stop consuming inflammatory foods, then the result wouldn't be that good. You will have to say a decisive no to the foods that are responsible for causing inflammation. The age-old saying 'prevention is better than cure' is absolutely true in this context.

Some of the ingredients to be avoided are:

Refined Sugar

Refined sugars are simply bad. They are devoid of nutrients and simply spike your blood sugar levels. You not only get extra calories that lead to faster weight gain but it can also cause suppression of white blood cell production. Inflammation can become a routine due to the damage caused by consuming excess refined sugar. A certain type of cancers, diabetes, and heart diseases have been linked with consumption of refined sugar. Sugar and salt are white poisons that must always be consumed with great restraint.

Saturated Fats

Saturated fats are already getting a lot of flak all over the world for the negative weight impact caused by them. But people generally ignore the other more dangerous aspect of saturated fats. They are pro-inflammatory and may promote systematic inflammation. Saturated fats may cause inflammation in the fat cells in your body. This will start a vicious cycle of inflammation. You can also come in the grip of various chronic illnesses. Keeping a strict control on the saturated fat intake is very important.

Trans Fats

You can measure them by any standard, and you'll always find that trans fats are off limits. Our body doesn't have the proper mechanism to process trans fats, and that's why they are always treated like a foreign object. Consumption of trans fats can trigger an inflammatory response that can also cause damage to the lining of blood vessels.

Trans fats will cause systematic inflammation and cause serious damage to your health. Delicacies like doughnuts, muffins, and margarine may look tempting, but they are inflammatory.

Refined Carbohydrates

The idea of sweetness without sugar and calories looked very tempting to the world. It became an instant craze giving birth to low-calorie diet drinks and no sugar added products. But, not everything that glitters is gold. Artificial sweeteners have raised the eyebrows of health agencies all over the world. These sweeteners can increase the risk of glucose intolerance. The gut microbiomes get affected, and it can lead to the development of type 2 diabetes. The destruction of good bacteria in your gut by these sweeteners has a serious inflammatory response. Always go by the golden rule that the natural is the best.

Gluten

Gluten in most of the refined flour bread is difficult to digest for our bodies. It can cause inflammation in the lining of the intestines. Your weight loss efforts would go in vain, and you can face several digestion issues along with inflammation. Getting gluten intolerance is also not a very far-fetched possibility. If you are trying to adopt an anti-inflammatory diet then staying away from gluten products is always a great idea.

Artificial ingredients

Anything that has been manufactured synthetically and isn't found freely in nature will interfere with your system. The same is true for artificial ingredients like MSG and several other tastemakers. They may add some taste to your food but prove to be very tasteless for your immune system. They can cause severe inflammation and cause damage to your health.

Vegetable oils

The use of vegetable oils has increased a lot in the past few decades and especially with the emergence of fast food chains they have become unavoidable. However, vegetable oils can cause serious damage to your health. These oils have a high percentage of harmful omega-6 fatty acids. High consumption of vegetable oils in the form of deep-fried items, chips, mayonnaise, and crackers can create a serious imbalance between the omega-3 fatty acids and omega-6 fatty acids. Ideally, the ratio should be 1:1 in our body, but it is several times more increasing the risk of inflammation. You must avoid using vegetable oils as much as possible.

Processed Meats

Meat and especially the red meat is difficult to digest. Our digestion system has to overtime to break all the proteins and nutrients. In addition to that, red meat is also high in saturated fats that aren't very good for the health. What makes it worse is the fact that most of the meat consumed these days is processed. It comes from large units where the animals are corn fed and also infused with antibiotics. This escalates the problem to a completely different level.

The consumption of meat should be minimized, and if consumed only grass-fed, antibiotic free animals should be eaten.

The bacterial toxins in the meat can trigger endotoxins in the blood. It has a high percentage of omega-6 fatty acids and increases the chances of inflammation.

Alcohol

Alcoholic beverages are a big reason of inflammation to the liver, gut, joints, tissues and the blood vessels. They increase the risk of heart diseases, cancer, and other issues related to your digestive system. Moderation is the key if you drink alcohol and it is best if you can avoid it.

Fast food

The dangers hidden in fast food is no secret to anyone. Yet, we choose to ignore it because we often think that we aren't eating much. It is a blatant lie to ourselves and a grave mistake. Any amount of fast food is bad and must be avoided. It is highly inflammatory, leads to obesity, digestive tract issues and host of other problems. There is a good reason it is called the 'junk food.'

Eliminating fast food from your diet will be the first constructive step towards an anti-inflammatory diet.

Conclusion

Thanks for making it through to the end of this book, let's hope it was informative and able to provide you with all of the tools you need to achieve your goals whatever they may be.

Health must be a priority for everyone as for achieving anything in life you need to be healthy. But, the fast-paced life the modern world has diverted our focus from a healthy body and mind to other things. Wrong dietary habits, lack of physical activity and stress lead to various health issues. They deprive you of enjoying your hard earned success. It is very important that you do not neglect your health at any stage and food plays a very important role in it.

Wrong food choices may spell trouble for you as they can trigger chronic inflammation. A system that is designed to work for your benefit starts working overtime and causes serious health issues. This is more dangerous than anything else as you consume food many times a day. It starts working as a slow poison for your body. You can get a number of health issues ranging from diabetes and heart diseases to cancer. This can be prevented if you follow a good diet. It doesn't ask you to do anything out of the ordinary. You only need to be careful about what to eat and what to leave.

This book tells you about the healthy things you should eat for stopping the development of chronic inflammation. Nature has provided scores of items that are very healthy and eliminate the risk of inflammation. This book has picked the best items from the list and presented them in front of you to consider in your diet. It explains the benefits you can reap by adopting a healthy anti-inflammatory diet.

You can stay healthy and enjoy the gifts of life in a better way if you adopt an anti-inflammatory diet. You have ample choices, and this diet will not deprive you of taste or delicacies. You only need to devote some time and intent to adopting this diet into your daily routine. It is important to remember that shortage of time is only an excuse we give to ourselves for not doing something. We can have all the time to ourselves if we want. In fact, this diet doesn't even ask you to take out a huge amount of time. So even that excuse is not very valid.

An anti-inflammatory diet will bring a positive change in your life. You will feel fresh, healthy and rejuvenated. You wouldn't have the guilt pangs that you get when you eat the wrong food. You will be able to manage your weight easily. You will also be able to stay away from unwanted medical issues if you follow a good anti-inflammatory diet.

The only thing you need to do is make up your mind and choose the right things to eat. Your reading of this part of the book already demonstrates a will to incorporate this change. It is the first constructive step that you have taken. Now, all you need to do is start eating the healthy food items mentioned in the book and feel the positive shift in your health parameters.

Finally, if you found this book useful in any way, a review on Amazon is always appreciated!

Other Books By Elizabeth Wells

Mediterranean Diet For Beginners
The Complete Guide To Lose Weight And Live Healthier Following The Mediterranean Lifestyle

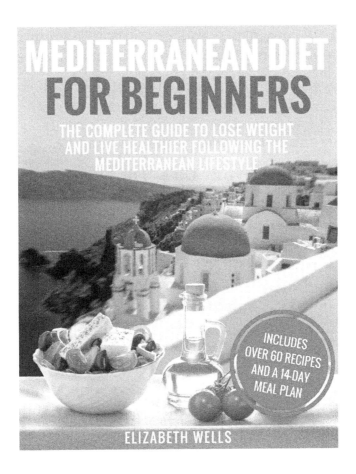

The Mediterranean Diet has been voted by many scientists as one of the healthiest diets in the world. The pure reality of this diet plan is that it isn't something to be considered as a short-term fad diet plan. It is a lifestyle that is loaded with healthy habits, great food, and a substantial amount of benefits, and it has been proven to help lose weight faster and achieve several other benefits like lower risk of heart disease and decreased risk of type 2 diabetes.

The Mediterranean Diet is based on the eating habits of people living in the Mediterranean region, and includes relatively high consumption of olive oil, vegetables and fruits and moderate consumption of fish, cheese, yogurt and other dairy products.

In this book you'll learn everything you need to know to lose weight, improve your overall health and experience the countless benefits of the Mediterranean lifestyle.

The Mediterranean Diet For Beginners Will Teach You:

- The Basics Of The Mediterranean Diet Plan
- How To Lose Weight The Mediterranean Way
- 11 Health Benefits You'll Get By Following The Mediterranean Lifestyle
- What You Should Eat And Drink - Explained
- How To Eat The Right Amounts Of Servings Using The Mediterranean Pyramid
- 5 Unhealthy Food Groups To Avoid
- A Complete 14-day Mediterranean Meal Plan
- 3 Healthy Alternatives To Common Unhealthy Foods
- Tips And Tricks For Eating Healthy Even When Eating Out
- A List Of Healthier (And Delicious) Choices To Order At The Most Famous Restaurants
- 60+ Mediterranean Diet Recipes For Tasty Breakfasts, Lunches, Sides, Dinners, Desserts, Snacks, Smoothies And Sauces
- And Much, Much More

And remember, the Mediterranean diet is not a restrictive eating style and even embraces food such as eggs, cheese, meat and some sweets – just in small amounts to savor and enjoy. The secret is to do as the Mediterranean people have done for centuries: eat healthy food, get walking and make exercise a part of your healthy routine, and if the moment comes, don't be leery of opening that bottle of rich cabernet you have been savoring for special occasions.

Some Mediterranean Diet Recipes You'll Find Inside The Book:

- Bento Lunchtime Delight
- Mediterranean Chicken Quinoa Bowl
- Mediterranean Tuna Antipasto Salad
- Greek Egg Frittata
- Herbed Mashed Potatoes with Greek Yogurt
- Marinated Olives & Feta
- Picnic Snack
- Hassel-back Caprese Chicken
- Salmon Rice Bowl
- Shrimp Scampi
- Cucumber Roll-Ups
- Cherries – Toasted Almonds and Ricotta

Enjoy your new lifestyle today!

"Mediterranean Diet For Beginners" by Elizabeth Wells is available at Amazon.

Keto Diet For Beginners
Complete Beginner's Guide To Lose Weight Fast And Live Healthier With Ketogenic Cooking

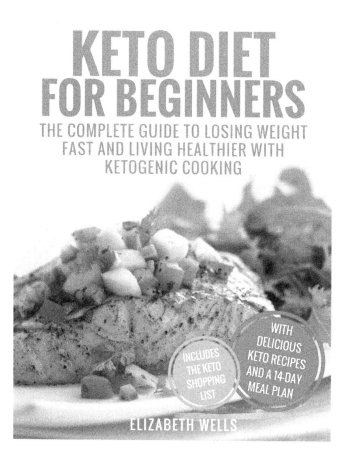

Would you like to lose weight and feel better without only eating salads? Have you already followed countless diets, without actually seeing any results? This one is different, and the results will speak for themselves.

The Ketogenic Diet, or Keto Diet, is a solid dieting program created back in 1924 by Dr. Russel Wilder and supported by many scientific studies. The Keto

Diet is not another diet that promises you everything and delivers you little to nothing! This dieting style lost popularity when some sketchy "lose weight effortlessly" diets came out some years ago, but it is now being acclaimed worldwide again, with famous people following it and new scientific studies being published.

The Keto Diet is based on this principle: your body usually gets energy from the carbs you eat and stores all the excess fats (think about love handles or belly fat). Most diets tell you to stop eating fats to lose weight, however there's a better way to do it.

Some types of fats are healthy and eating them more, while also reducing your intake of carbs, will help you lose weight faster. In fact, if you start eating low carb and high fat your body will use the fats instead of the carbohydrates to produce energy, without actually storing them.

This way, your body will naturally burn fats for you, just by eating the right foods. And the best part is ketogenic foods actually taste really good. Imagine how ketogenic cooking will improve your shape and overall health.

"Once you have been on the ketogenic diet for a few weeks and begun to experience its benefits you will never want to go back to high-carb eating. After all, ketosis is the body's natural state. It's how we were designed to live."

Following this diet is easy when you have the right help. That's why this book will teach you **everything you need to know about the keto diet** to help you lose weight fast and feel better, without being too tricky or complicated. You'll learn exactly what to eat, what to avoid, what recipes to cook, what to store in your pantry to follow the keto diet correctly and start improving your health right now.

Some benefits you'll get by going keto:

- Lose Weight Fast And In A Natural Way
- Feel Better, Both Mentally And Physically
- Eat Healthy Foods That Actually Taste Good
- Have A Healthy, Younger Looking Skin
- Feel Full Of Energy All Day Long
- Lower Your Triglyceride Levels To Prevent Heart Attacks
- Eat Foods That Won't Leave You Hungry All Day
- Improve Your Physical Performance
- Lower Your Cancer Risk
- And Much, Much More

In this book you'll learn:

- What Is The Ketogenic Diet and How It Works
- All The Real Benefits Of The Ketogenic Diet
- A Complete 14-day Keto Meal Plan To Successfully Go Keto
- 20+ Delicious Keto Recipes For Breakfast, Lunch And Dinner
- A List Of Keto Friendly Foods To Store In Your Pantry
- The Complete Keto Shopping List To Fill Your Cart With Healthy Foods
- How To Know If You Shouldn't Follow This Diet
- Simple Tips And Tricks To Stay Keto While Travelling
- How To Stay On The Keto Diet Through The

Holidays
- And Much More

Start improving your health today!

"Keto Diet For Beginners" by Elizabeth Wells is available at Amazon.

ELIZABETH WELLS

Keto Pressure Cooker
101 Delicious Ketogenic Recipes For The Electric Pressure Cooker To Lose Weight Fast And Live Healthier

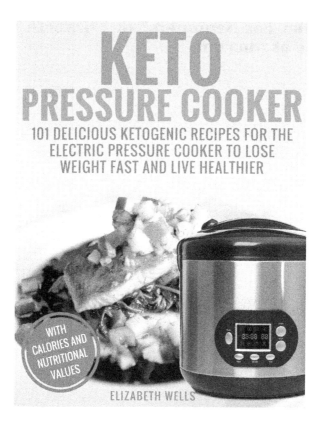

If you love the ketogenic diet and would like to cook dishes using your electric pressure cooker this book is for you. Cooking keto using an electric pressure cooker will help you save time and money without losing the countless benefits of a high fat, low carb diet.

In this cookbook, you'll find 101 mouthwatering ketogenic recipes for every meal time, breakfast, lunch, dinner, sides and desserts. All the recipes include comprehensive instructions and nutritional values, allowing you to know the amount of calories, fats, carbohydrates and proteins contained in each dish.

With the help of these recipes you will easily transition toward a healthier lifestyle.

Some recipes you'll find:
- Korean Steamed Eggs
- Ham And Pepper Fritatta
- Italian Sausage Kale Soup
- Creamy Cauliflower Chowder
- Cream Of Mushroom
- Shredded Chicken
- Green Beans And Bacon
- Prosciutto Wrapped-asparagus
- Coconut Milk Shrimp
- Salmon With Orange Ginger Sauce
- Garlic Cuban Pork
- Garlic And Parmesan Asparagus
- Pumpkin Cheesecake
- Chocolate Mousse
- Coconut Almond Cake
- Chocolate Cheesecake
- And Much More

Enjoy these keto dishes today!

"Keto Pressure Cooker" by Elizabeth Wells is available at Amazon.

ELIZABETH WELLS

Keto Slow Cooker
101 Delicious Ketogenic Recipes For The Slow Cooker To Lose Weight Fast And Live Healthier

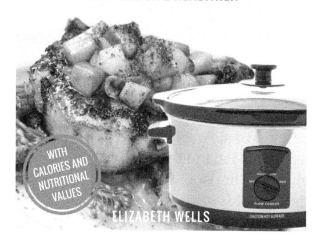

Are you on a ketogenic diet and would love to cook using your slow cooker? Imagine putting a bunch of ingredients in your slow cooker before going to work and coming home to a delicious keto approved meal.

In this cookbook, you'll find 101 delicious ketogenic recipes you can easily cook with your slow cooker. Just follow the simple steps, put all the ingredients in, and let the slow cooker do the rest. You'll discover recipes for chilis, soups, stews, beef meals, poultry and pork dishes, desserts and other tasty treats that will help you save time without losing the countless benefits of a high fat, low carb diet.

All the recipes include step-by-step instructions and nutritional values, allowing you to know the amount of calories, fats, carbohydrates and proteins contained in each dish. And remember, you don't have to spend your entire day in the kitchen to cook healthy dishes.

Some recipes you'll find:
- Chicken Chorizo Soup
- Hare Stew
- BBQ Pulled Beef
- Balsamic Chicken Thighs
- Cuban Ropa Vieja
- Cranberry Pork Roast
- Poached Salmon
- Zucchini Bread
- Chile Verde
- Summertime Veggies
- Jamaican Jerk Roast
- Raspberry Coconut Cake
- Lemon Frosted Cake
- Grain-Free Granola
- And Much More

Enjoy your new recipes today!

"Keto Slow Cooker" by Elizabeth Wells is available at Amazon.

Keto Diet For Beginners
The Step By Step Guide For Beginners To Lose Weight Fast And Live Healthier With The Ketogenic Diet

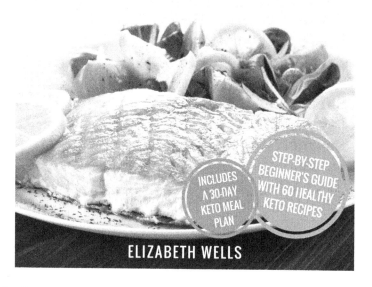

Let's face it, so many people are already in love with this high-fat, low carb diet these days, but there's so much information out there that it can be very overwhelming to figure out how to follow the ketogenic diet without making the most common mistakes.

If you're interested in the keto diet, but don't know where to start, look no further. In this beginner's guide you'll find everything you need to know to start a keto diet and be successful on your dieting journey.

This book will take you step by step through the fundamental principles of the keto diet, will answer all the most common questions and will teach you what foods to eat and what to avoid without being too complicated or overwhelming. After reading this book, you will be well on your way to entering the state known as "ketosis" and jump-starting your new weight loss regimen on the Keto lifestyle.

In this guide you'll find:
- A Step-by-step Process To Start A Keto Diet The Right Way
- History And Fundamental Principles Of The Keto Diet
- How The Ketogenic Diet Works And What You Need To Start Today
- A 30-day Meal Plan Template To Guide You With All The Recipes You Need
- 60 Healthy Ketogenic Recipes For Healthy Breakfast, Lunch, Dinner, Desserts, Snacks And Salads
- A Complete List Of Foods You Should And Shouldn't Eat
- All The Health Benefits You'll Get By Going Keto
- How To Avoid The Common Mistakes All Beginners Make While Starting The Keto Diet
- Ketogenic FAQs: Answers To All The Most Common Questions About The Ketogenic Diet

You will learn all about ketogenic, fasting, weight

loss, and how a low-carb, high-protein diet can change your life mentally, physically, and even emotionally. This book covers its origins as a treatment for epilepsy to all the health problems we face in today's highly processed, fast food world, and how this all contributes to our health. Once you decide to begin a ketogenic diet you will be helping yourself against obesity, diabetes, inflammatory diseases, heart health, curbing dementia, and so much more!

You'll learn how to start the Keto diet successfully with a step-by-step process on how to begin, as well as an extensive list of foods that can and cannot be eaten, so you will be able to know from the start exactly what you should be eating. You'll also find a 30-day meal planning guide along with all the recipes so you can begin planning and hop right away, no need to research for recipes!

Some recipes you'll find in this book:
- Garlic Cedar Plank Salmon
- Prosciutto Wrapped Asparagus
- Tuna Lettuce Wrap With Avocado Yogurt Dressing
- Chicken and Cilantro Salad
- Grilled Salmon with Avocado Bruschetta
- Steak With Balsamic Tomatoes
- California Spicy Crab Stuffed Avocado
- Chicken Pesto Bake
- Zucchini Rolls
- Sausage Stuffed Zucchini with Mozzarella Cheese
- Steak Kebabs with Chimichurri
- Flourless Chocolate Keto Brownies
- Cinnamon Pecan Bars

- Raspberry Lemon Cupcakes
- And Much More

And the best part is, these recipes actually taste good, because remember, being on a diet doesn't have to mean eating flavorless food.

Start the Keto Diet today!

"Keto Diet For Beginners" by Elizabeth Wells is available at Amazon.

Keto Diet
Complete Beginner's Guide To Lose Weight Fast And Live Healthier With Ketogenic Cooking

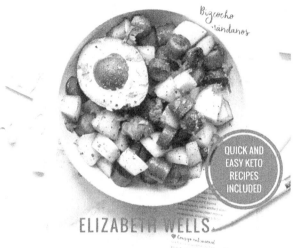

Have you already tried every known diet without seeing any results? Are you willing to lose weight and improve your health but don't want to quit eating some of your loved dishes?

You've come to the right place. The Ketogenic Diet is a popular dieting program that has been around for decades. The Keto Diet is not another fad regime that promises you everything and delivers you little to nothing! This dieting style has been created by Dr. Russell Wilder back in 1924 and is proven and supported by many scientific studies. It lost popularity when some fad "lose weight quick" diets came out some decades ago.

Recently it is being rediscovered and is already acclaimed worldwide. The Keto Diet is well known for being a low carb diet, where the body produces ketones instead of glucose to be used as energy. This will help it burn fats to produce energy without storing them and will drastically reduce the amount of weight you accumulate.

"Eating high fat and low carb offers many health, weight loss, physical and mental performance benefits."

You don't have to quit eating fats to lose weight. You'll still be able to enjoy food that actually tastes good and makes you happy.

In this book you'll learn how the Keto Diet works and how you can start improving your health right now by cooking delicious dishes.

These are some of the benefits you'll get:

- Lose weight naturally and easily
- Feel well, both mentally and physically
- Keep your skin younger looking
- Eat healthy foods you actually like
- Satisfy your appetite without remaining hungry all day
- Achieve a lower blood pressure
- Prevent heart attacks by lowering your triglyceride levels
- Increase your energy and improve your physical performance
- Lower your cancer risk

- And much more

Following this diet without any help can be complex, especially if you're a beginner. That's why this book aims to teach you everything you need to know to improve your eating habits and your life, without being too tricky or complicated.

In this book you'll learn:

- What is the Ketogenic Diet
- What You Should Eat (And What You Shouldn't)
- 43 Recommended Foods (with calories, grams of carbs, proteins and fats contained)
- How To Follow The Keto Diet Correctly (Most People Get This Wrong)
- 3 Signs That You've Reached Ketosis
- The Benefits Of Going Keto
- 50 Quick And Easy To Cook Keto Recipes
- And much more

What are you waiting for? Start eating healthier today!

"Keto Diet" by Elizabeth Wells is available at Amazon.

Keto Meal Prep
Complete Beginner's Guide To Save Time And Eat Healthier With Batch Cooking For The Ketogenic Diet

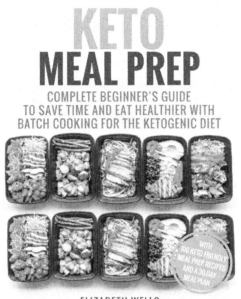

If you're one of the thousands of people on a ketogenic diet you already know and love all its benefits and the amount of energy a low-carb, high-fat diet can give you. Unfortunately, cooking healthy dishes usually takes time, and not everyone can spend 3+ hours in the kitchen every day to cook for breakfast, lunch and dinner. If you're looking for a way to save time while still eating delicious keto approved dishes, this book is for you.

Learning how to plan and cook your meals in advance is one of the best things that you can do. Meal prepping, also known as batch cooking, helps you stay on the ketogenic diet, makes it easy to save time during the week, keeps you away from your temptations, and can even save you a lot of money. And when you combine the ketogenic diet with your meal prepping goals, you are going to lose weight and feel great in no time.

This guidebook is going to provide you with all the tools that you need to get started with meal prepping on the ketogenic diet.

In this guidebook you'll learn:
- The Basic Principles Of The Ketogenic Diet
- The Right Way To Start Meal Prepping Today
- How To Avoid The Common Mistakes Made By Meal Prepping Beginners
- 100 Keto Friendly Meal Prep Recipes For Easy Breakfasts, Lunches And Dinners, Snacks And Desserts
- A Complete 30-day Meal Plan To Keep You On Your Goals
- And Much More

Some of the meal prep recipes you'll find:
- Keto Monkey Bread
- Roast Beef Cups
- Pork Salad
- Baked Chicken Nuggets
- Pumpkin Soup
- Super Green Soup
- Beef Stew
- Chocolate and Peanut Butter Muffins
- Blender pancakes
- Butter Coffee
- Walnut Bites
- Smoked Salmon and Dill Spread
- Lime and Coconut Fat Bombs
- Low Carb Bars

- Avocado Tropical Treat
- Keto Lava Cake
- And Many Other Recipes

Save time and eat healthier with meal prepping on a ketogenic diet

"Keto Meal Prep" by Elizabeth Wells is available at Amazon.

Meal Prep Guide
Discover How To Lose Weight, Spend Less Time In The Kitchen And Eat Healthier With Meal Prepping

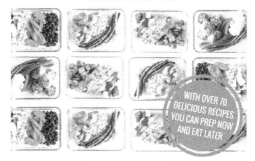

Do you work a full-time job or just have a busy lifestyle and find it difficult to prepare a healthy meal every day?

Cooking takes time, and with our busy lives not everybody can spend hours in the kitchen everyday. Meal prepping, also known as batch cooking, is the definitive solution to this problem. By learning how to cook your meals in advance and store them safely you'll be able to easily save time (and money) while still eating healthy, homemade food.

In this book you'll learn all the basics you need to know to start meal prepping your food and store it safely. You'll also find over 70 delicious recipes suitable for meal prepping that will teach you how to cook delicious dishes for your breakfasts, dinners, lunches, desserts, and lunch boxes.

You'll learn:

- How To Save Time And Cook Healthy Dishes With Meal Prepping
- The Meal Prep Method: How To Prep And Safely Store Eggs, Meat, Grains And Fruits
- 70+ Delicious Recipes To Save Time And Cook Healthy Dishes For Breakfast, Lunch, Dinner And Dessert.
- One-Serving Smoothie Recipes For Healthy Snacks To Enjoy At Any Time Of The Day
- And Much More

With this unique collection of recipes, you will be able to stock your refrigerator with tasty meals and snacks to please everyone in your household.

Here are some recipes you'll find inside the book:

- Mexican Breakfast Taquitos
- Chickpea & Butternut Fajitas
- Apple Butternut Squash Soup
- Egg Cups
- Black Bean & Sweet Potato Salad
- Southwestern Sweet Potato Lentil Jar Salad
- Cilantro Lime Chicken & Cauliflower Rice
- Green Tropical Bowl
- Almond Butter - Brown Rice Crispy Treats
- Banana Strawberry & Green Smoothie

Stop eating junk food just because you don't have enough time to cook healthy.

Start meal prepping today!

"Meal Prep Guide" by Elizabeth Wells is available at Amazon.

Ketogenic Diet Guide For Beginners:

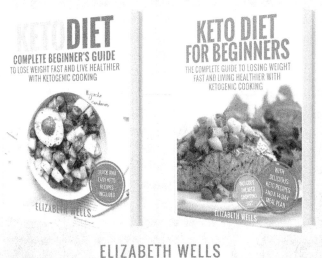

"Ketogenic Diet Guide For Beginners" by Elizabeth Wells is available at Amazon.

Made in the USA
Middletown, DE
13 September 2020